UNDERSTANDING TYPE 2 DIABETES AND HIGH BLOOD PRESSURE 2 BOOKS IN 1

SIMPLE STEPS TO AVOID COMPLICATIONS, REDUCE MEDICAL EXPENSES, DECREASE STRESS, AND LIVE A HEALTHY & PROACTIVE LIFE

DR. ASHLEY SULLIVAN, PHARMD, RPH, MBA

Copyright © 2023 by Dr. Ashley Sullivan, PharmD, RPh, MBA. All rights reserved.

The content contained within this book may not be reproduced, duplicated, or transmitted without direct written permission from the author or the publisher.

Under no circumstances will any blame or legal responsibility be held against the publisher, or author, for any damages, reparation, or monetary loss due to the information contained within this book, either directly or indirectly.

Legal Notice:

This book is copyright protected. It is only for personal use. You cannot amend, distribute, sell, use, quote, or paraphrase any part, or the content within this book, without the consent of the author or publisher.

Disclaimer Notice:

Please note the information contained within this document is for educational and entertainment purposes only. All effort has been executed to present accurate, up-to-date, reliable, and complete information. No warranties of any kind are declared or implied. Readers acknowledge that the author is not engaged in the rendering of legal, financial, medical, or professional advice. The content within this book has been derived from various sources. Please consult a licensed professional before attempting any techniques outlined in this book.

By reading this document, the reader agrees that under no circumstances is the author responsible for any losses, direct or indirect, that are incurred as a result of the use of the information contained within this document, including, but not limited to, errors, omissions, or inaccuracies.

TABLE OF CONTENTS

UNDERSTANDING TYPE 2 DIABETES

Introduction	7
1. What is Type 2 Diabetes?	13
2. Understanding Insulin and Blood Sugar	33
3. The Causes and Prevention of Diabetes	53
4. Treatment Options for Diabetes	67
5. Managing Diabetes Through Diet	87
6. Exercise and Physical Activity for Diabetes Management	113
7. Managing Type 2 Diabetes Complications	123
8. The Role of Medications in Type 2 Diabetes Management	135
9. Mental Health and Emotional Well-Being with Diabetes	153
10. Advocating for Your Health with Type 2 Diabetes	165
Conclusion	179
Glossary	183
References	187

UNDERSTANDING HIGH BLOOD PRESSURE

Introduction	205
1. Under Pressure	213
2. What Puts You at Risk for High Blood Pressure?	241
3. Medications for Managing High Blood Pressure	251
4. Healthy Food for a Happy Heart	291
5. Move It and Lose It	315

6. Rest and Relaxation	335
7. Kicking Bad Habits	353
8. Beyond Medications	365
9. The Hidden Dangers	391
10. Stay on Top of Your Health	407
Conclusion	423
References	427

UNDERSTANDING TYPE 2 DIABETES

SIMPLE STEPS TO AVOID COMPLICATIONS, REDUCE MEDICAL EXPENSES, DECREASE STRESS, AND LIVE A HEALTHY & PROACTIVE LIFE

INTRODUCTION

According to the Centers for Disease Control and Prevention (CDC), over 34 million Americans have diabetes. 90 to 95% of those cases are type 2 diabetes.

Whether you've recently been diagnosed with type 2 diabetes or you've been living with it for many years, keeping your blood sugar under control can be an overwhelming, lonely experience.

I say this as someone who has worked in the medical field for many years. I have seen firsthand the frustration my patients have when they go to the pharmacy to pick up insulin or testing supplies and they have high costs even with insurance. I have seen the fear in their eyes when they've been told that they're at risk for vision problems or kidney disease. I sense the anxiety they're feeling, and my heart goes out to everyone who has been affected by this disease.

But know this - you are not alone.

Diabetes is incredibly common, as you can see from the statistic above, but it's also important to note that you are *not* just a statistic. You are a person. And I see you.

As someone with diabetes, you may be faced with a laundry list of symptoms and potential complications. Your gut instinct might be to turn to your doctor for advice, but the reality is that not all of us have doctors whom we feel like we can confide in. There are so many barriers to receiving proper treatment, and it is tough to know what steps to take.

If you or someone you love has recently been diagnosed with type 2 diabetes, it is understandable that you may feel overwhelmed and unsure of where to start. Type 2 diabetes is a chronic condition that affects millions of people worldwide and managing it can be challenging.

As you already know, type 2 diabetes is a condition where the body either does not produce enough insulin or is not able to use insulin effectively. Insulin is a hormone that is responsible for regulating blood sugar levels in the body.

Common symptoms of type 2 diabetes include frequent urination, excessive thirst, fatigue, and blurred vision. Understanding these symptoms and how they relate to the condition can help you manage it better, but as someone who has the disease, you might not fully understand how these specific symptoms will affect you specifically - after all, everybody is different.

One of the biggest challenges of managing type 2 diabetes is controlling blood sugar levels, which can fluctuate based on numerous factors such as diet, exercise, stress, and medication.

Monitoring your blood sugar levels regularly can provide insight into how these factors affect your body, but again, it is a tough balance to strike between proper nutrition, exercise, stress, and medication. Often, the recommendations given to us by medical professionals are generalized - they are not customized to your unique situation.

Sure, you should be limiting stress in your day-to-day life. But you are the parent of three kids under five years old, you have a demanding 40-hour-a-week job, and various life stressors on top of that - stressors you cannot necessarily avoid. You need advice that is tailored to your unique situation.

To make matters worse, there are many stressful factors that complicate this disease. We know that people with type 2 diabetes are at risk for a range of complications, including nerve damage, vision problems, kidney disease, and heart disease. But there is a good chance you don't want to live in constant fear of those progressive symptoms.

The cost of managing type 2 diabetes can be high, including regular doctor visits, medications, and medical devices such as glucose meters and insulin pumps. Even if you have excellent insurance, it is tough to predict what will and won't be covered.

It is safe to say that receiving a diagnosis of type 2 diabetes can be emotionally challenging - and it can impact your mental health and self-esteem.

The fear of these complications and potential expenses can be overwhelming and cause anxiety, but it is important to remember that with proper management, these risks can be significantly reduced. Regular check-ups with your doctor and taking medications as prescribed can help prevent complications from worsening. Having the right information and a basic knowledge of what you are up against is also helpful.

That is where I come in.

Managing type 2 diabetes can be a lonely experience, and you could benefit from emotional and social support to help you stay motivated and positive. I want to help alleviate some of your emotional burden by teaching you everything you need to know about how to manage your diabetes so you can live a fulfilling, happy, and stress-free life (or at least, somewhat stress-free!) life.

I know that a diagnosis of type 2 diabetes comes with a lot of *really* big feelings. You might be angry that others misunderstand your condition or angry at presumptions that your diabetes was caused by poor lifestyle decisions you made.

You might feel frustrated or helpless, upset that your symptoms are interfering with your daily life. You might be unsure of how you are going to afford next month's medications or doctors' appointments. You might feel judged or criticized by others. You might feel like you are just going through the motions, trying to get from one day to the next, rather than being able to enjoy life.

Again. You are not alone. These feelings are normal, and I want to help you work through them.

Proper education is the first step in any journey, and that is where this book comes in. If you want to have the confidence you need to manage your diabetes, you need to understand everything there is to know about it. You need to understand the best recommendations for:

- Stress management
- Nutrition and exercise
- Lifestyle adjustments and essential diet control tips as a first line of defense to manage your condition
- Managing your blood sugar levels
- Medication treatment options

I'll give you a complete review of the technology, trends, and modern science around the condition - no more outdated pamphlets from the waiting room of your doctor's office.

And most importantly, I'll give you the knowledge and empowerment you need to advocate for yourself - and for a person-centered approach to managing your condition. There is a glossary of medical terms at the end of the book before the references. Citations follow the end of the book, although a lot of the information presented is from my professional education and work experience.

Whether your goal is to be able to manage your symptoms without medication or just to reduce your symptoms, this book is for you.

I did not come by this knowledge overnight. As I mentioned earlier, I have worked for several years in the medical field, and I've worked closely with dozens of patients just like you. I know where you are coming from. I know how hard this is. And I want to help you better understand diabetes.

Are you ready to get started? Let us take a deep dive into type 2 diabetes - and let's get you on the track toward a brighter, more empowered future.

1

WHAT IS TYPE 2 DIABETES?

Diabetes is a chronic condition that affects millions of people around the world. According to the 2020 National Diabetes Statistics Report, around 34.2 million people in the United States have diabetes, which accounts for 10.5% of the US population. Diabetes is a disease that impacts the way the body processes blood sugar or glucose. Broadly speaking, there are two types of diabetes: type 1 and type 2. This book will dive into type 2 diabetes, but it is important to note that there are many commonalities shared between the two.

WHAT IS TYPE 2 DIABETES?

Type 2 Diabetes is a chronic condition that occurs when your body becomes resistant to insulin, or when the pancreas produces inadequate insulin. Insulin is a hormone that regulates blood sugar, and without it, glucose surges in your bloodstream and can cause serious problems.

Over time, high levels of glucose in the blood can lead to severe complications such as neuropathy (nerve pain), blindness, and kidney problems. Type 2 Diabetes is the most diagnosed type of diabetes, with nearly 90% of the diabetes cases being Type 2 in the US.

What Causes Type 2 Diabetes?

Type 2 diabetes is caused by a combination of genetic and environmental factors. Individuals with a family history of the disease are more likely to develop it.

Obesity, a sedentary lifestyle, and poor dietary habits also increase the risk of developing type 2 diabetes. People with metabolic syndrome, a condition that includes high blood pressure and elevated cholesterol levels, are also at risk of developing type 2 diabetes.

Regardless of the cause, type 2 diabetes occurs when the body becomes resistant to insulin or when the pancreas fails to produce enough insulin, a hormone that regulates blood sugar levels.

Is Type 2 Diabetes Serious?

You probably already know this, but diabetes can be serious if left untreated. High levels of glucose in the blood can cause damage to various organs and lead to complications such as blindness, kidney disease, nerve damage, heart disease, and stroke.

Can Type 2 Diabetes Be Cured?

While type 2 diabetes cannot be cured, it can be managed with proper treatment and lifestyle changes. The goal of treatment is to keep blood sugar levels in the target range to prevent complications.

Treatment may involve medications such as metformin, controlling blood pressure and cholesterol levels, and regular exercise and weight loss. In some cases, bariatric surgery may be considered if obesity is an underlying issue related to the diagnosis of diabetes.

Many people can reduce their medications if they make lifestyle changes to help control their blood glucose levels. You should always work with your medical provider when making changes and communicate your goals for treatment.

Type 2 Diabetes Treatment Options

The treatment for type 2 diabetes may vary depending on an individual's unique needs. The treatment plan may include medications that help lower blood sugar levels and improve insulin sensitivity, such as metformin, sulfonylureas (glipizide, glimepiride, glyburide), or thiazolidinediones (pioglitazone). These options are discussed further into the book.

Perhaps more importantly, lifestyle changes such as weight loss, regular exercise, and healthy eating can help manage blood sugar, blood pressure, and cholesterol.

It is essential to work closely with a healthcare provider to develop a personalized treatment plan that works best for you. In this book, I will walk you through some potential treatment options that you may find effective and helpful.

WHY ARE SO MANY PEOPLE AFFECTED?

In the United States alone, more than 34 million people have diabetes, and millions of others are at risk of developing the disease. Type 2 diabetes is on the rise, and several factors contribute to this alarming trend.

Obesity

The first and most significant factor contributing to the rise in type 2 diabetes is obesity.

In the US, obesity has been on the increase over the past 15 years, and there has been an increase in diabetes rates to correspond with that rise. There are a few reasons for this, but the most significant to note is that obesity increases insulin resistance, which leads to high levels of glucose in the blood, leading to diabetes.

Lack of Physical Activity

Lack of physical activity is another contributing factor to the rise in type 2 diabetes. Our lifestyle has become increasingly sedentary, with a lot of time spent in front of screens. This means that exercise is not prioritized, and this lack of physical activity leads to weight gain and other health problems, including diabetes.

There is one story I'd like to mention here to illustrate the huge impact that physical activity has on diabetes. One man, Roger Hare, was diagnosed with type-2 diabetes in 2019. He told his story to a WebMD reporter shortly after his diagnosis. Like most people, he faced a variety of emotions upon hearing that he had diabetes. He was angry, panicked, and confused. He thought the world was coming to an end. However, he acted quickly, putting a plan together to drop some weight.

Although medication and nutrition played a big part in his weight loss (and reduction in diabetes symptoms), Hare noted the extreme importance of being active, stating, "Exercise plays a big role. I go to the gym two or three times a week for cardio and strength training. I normally start with 15-20 minutes on the treadmill. Then I will do some weightlifting and floor exercises. I cool down with another 10-15 minutes on the treadmill."

While it has not always been easy, he lost 40 pounds and dropped his A1C by more than 6 points. That is remarkable!

Dietary Changes

Dietary changes are also responsible for the increase in type 2 diabetes.

We are far more likely to eat foods that are high in sugar (even those that are not necessarily desserts - did you know that store-bought tomato sauce has a whopping 10 grams of sugar?). Carbonated drinks, packaged ready-to-eat foods, and fried foods, are all common factors leading to chronic inflammation and diabetes as well.

Awareness & Changes in Diagnostic Criteria

Awareness also plays a role in the rise of type 2 diabetes. There has been an increase in awareness regarding the health effects of diabetes and the importance of regular check-ups.

People are getting evaluated for diabetes earlier. That is a good thing, since it means that early detection is being prioritized and that people are taking the necessary measures to prevent the disease, but it also results in higher rates of diabetes being reported.

Doctors are now able to recommend exercises and dietary changes not just for people who have diabetes, but also those with prediabetes, which is the stage in which blood sugar levels are elevated, but not at the level of "full-blown" diabetes. There are about 96 million people in the US (aged

18 years or older) who have prediabetes. This is estimated to be around 38% of the population.

There are new tests available for diabetes as well. A new blood test, HbA1C, makes it possible to diagnose diabetes without the need for fasting for 12 hours. It is much more reliable and effective at diagnosing diabetes early on, especially in younger people.

Aging Population

Finally, the aging population is a contributing factor to the rise in type 2 diabetes. As we age, our body's ability to use insulin decreases, increasing the risk of developing diabetes.

With the baby-boomer generation reaching retirement age, there has been a corresponding (and expected) surge in diabetes cases among older adults.

THE HISTORY BEHIND TYPE 2 DIABETES

Now that you know what diabetes is and why it has become more common, let's take a closer look at the history behind the disease. Understanding our history is the best way to make smart, informed decisions in the future.

Believe it or not, the history of diabetes dates back to ancient times when it was described by physicians as a mysterious disease that caused frequent urination and emaciation (thin and weak).

The first recorded symptoms of diabetes were documented in 1552 B.C. by Hesy-Ra, an Egyptian physician who observed excessive urination as a key symptom of this befuddling disease that caused emaciation.

However, it was not until centuries later that physicians started to gain a better understanding of this condition. In 150 AD, the Greek doctor Arateus described diabetes as "the melting down of flesh and limbs into urine," thus highlighting the connection between sugar in urine and diabetes.

During the Middle Ages, a group of people began to diagnose diabetes. The way they did this was not with any fancy diagnostic test, but simply by tasting the urine of people who were believed to have diabetes. If the urine tasted sweet, the patient was diagnosed with diabetes. This group of people was known as "water tasters," and this is how diabetes was diagnosed for many centuries.

In 1675, the word "mellitus," which translates to honey, was added to the name "diabetes," which itself translated to the word "siphon." This was done to acknowledge the sweet, honey-like taste of the patient's urine. Believe it or not, it wasn't until later, in the 1800s, that scientists invented chemical tests to detect the presence of sugar in urine, making the diagnosis process much simpler (and not so unappetizing).

However, it was even earlier than that when physicians discovered that dietary changes could help manage diabetes.

They recommended that their patients eat only the fat and meat of animals or consume substantial amounts of sugar. Now we know how damaging sugar is to our body and how much it contributes to the development of diabetes, but back then they did not understand diabetes.

During the Franco-Prussian War of the early 1870s, a French physician Apollinaire Bouchardat noted that the symptoms of his diabetic patients showed a dramatic improvement. This was due to the cause of food rationing related to the war. As a result, Bouchardat created individualized diets that served as a core component of diabetes treatments.

In the early 1900s, fad diets became popular as treatments for diabetes. The "oat cure," "potato therapy," and the "starvation diet" were the most famous diets of the time. The oat cure involved consuming substantial amounts of oatmeal, while the potato therapy revolved around eating only potatoes for several days.

The starvation diet, on the other hand, involved severely restricting calories to induce weight loss. While these diets may have helped some diabetes patients temporarily, they were not sustainable and often did more harm than good.

In 1916, Boston scientist Elliott Joslin published *The Treatment of Diabetes Mellitus*, a textbook that established him as one of the world's leading diabetes experts. In his book, Joslin said that a fasting diet, when combined with physical activity, could reduce the mortality risk for diabetes patients.

This was a significant milestone in the development of diabetes management and the way we treat diabetes today.

Despite all these advances and research, before the discovery of insulin, diabetes almost always resulted in premature death. Insulin was discovered and first used in 1889 when Oskar Minkowski and Joseph von Mering found that the removal of a dog's pancreas could synthetically induce diabetes.

Then, in the 1920s, scientists discovered insulin, a hormone produced by the pancreas that is necessary to regulate blood sugar levels. As you might expect, this breakthrough discovery was an absolute game-changer in the treatment of diabetes. People with diabetes, who were once condemned to a life of extreme diets and constant monitoring, could now manage their condition with regular insulin injections.

Today, diabetes is still a major health concern, but of course, it's much more well-understood. People aged 40 and above are at the highest risk. However, recent studies show that young adults ages 18-34 are also at risk. In fact, the number of young adults being diagnosed with diabetes is on the rise. Your risk is higher if you are African Caribbean, Black African, or South Asian - or if you're male.

While it's important to note that while certain age groups and demographics are at a higher risk, diabetes can affect anyone at any age. It is also not an issue that's exclusive to the US. While there are 338 million people with diabetes in the United States as of 2023, there are more than a billion people each in China and India with the disease.

Let me say it again, as if these statistics do not demonstrate it well enough - you're not alone! The good news is that there are more researchers devoted to studying diabetes now, in 2023, than ever before and lots of good things are happening.

WHAT ARE THE RISK FACTORS FOR DIABETES?

Next, you might be wondering what makes you more likely to develop diabetes. While there are always outliers, there are a few common risk factors present in most cases of diagnosed diabetes.

Again, one significant risk factor for diabetes is weight. Being overweight or obese is a primary risk factor for developing type 2 diabetes. The more excess body fat you carry, particularly around your waistline, the more likely you are to develop diabetes.

It is so important to maintain a healthy weight to reduce your risk of developing diabetes. Regular exercise and a healthy diet can help you achieve this.

Another crucial factor to consider is inactivity. Living a sedentary lifestyle can increase your risk of developing diabetes, irrespective of your weight. Physical activity can help control your weight, improve glucose utilization, and increase your cells' insulin sensitivity.

Therefore, finding ways to get active, whether through exercise, walking, or other physical activities (or a combination, like our story of Roger Hare from above), can help reduce your risk of developing diabetes.

Family history is another significant factor to consider. People who have immediate family members with type 2 diabetes are at a higher risk of developing the condition. Therefore, regularly checking your blood sugar levels and having a conversation with your doctor about your family history can help diagnose and manage the condition early.

Other risk factors include age, cholesterol levels, prediabetes, and pregnancy-related risks. As you age, your risk for developing diabetes increases, particularly if you are over 35 years old.

Low levels of high-density lipoprotein (HDL), or "good" cholesterol, and elevated levels of triglycerides can also increase your risk of diabetes. Having prediabetes or a previous history of gestational diabetes or giving birth to a baby weighing more than nine pounds can also make you more susceptible to diabetes as well.

This is a risk factor that is seldom talked about - childbirth. In fact, one story of a diabetes patient, Jenn, as reported to The Johns Hopkins Patient Guide to Diabetes, highlights this well. Jenn was diagnosed with gestational diabetes for each one of her three pregnancies (usually in the third trimester). Even though Jenn is still at risk of developing adult onset type 2 diabetes was able to manage her condition by diet alone while she was pregnant, and it went away after she delivered each of her babies.

Smoking is also a risk factor of diabetes. People who smoke cigarettes are 30% - 40% more likely to develop type 2 diabetes than people who do not smoke. Nicotine can contribute to cells having a decreased response to insulin, resulting in elevated levels of glucose in the blood.

WHAT ARE THE MOST COMMON DIABETES SYMPTOMS?

One of the key aspects of managing type 2 diabetes is being aware of the symptoms. You may have some or all of these, but knowing about each of them is key to managing the condition successfully.

- **Increased thirst:** Do you feel like you are always reaching for a drink? Excessive thirst is one of the most common symptoms of diabetes. When your blood sugar levels rise, your body tries to get rid of the excess sugar by flushing it out through urine, but this can leave you dehydrated.
- **Frequent urination:** If you are suddenly finding yourself making more trips to the bathroom than usual, it could be another sign of diabetes. High

blood sugar levels can cause your kidneys to work overtime, trying to filter out the excess sugar. This can lead to more frequent trips to the bathroom, especially at night.

- **Increased hunger:** Constant hunger, even after eating, is another common symptom of diabetes. When your body cannot get the glucose it needs from food, it goes into overdrive looking for more fuel, which can result in increased hunger and food cravings.
- **Unintended weight loss**: Losing weight without trying might sound like a dream for some, but when it happens suddenly and without explanation, it can be a cause for concern (especially if you have that elevated appetite we mentioned earlier). In some people with diabetes, the body may start burning fat and muscle for energy instead of glucose, leading to unintentional weight loss.
- **Fatigue**: Diabetes can make you feel more fatigued than usual, because your body can't extract enough glucose from the food you eat for energy. This can leave you feeling depleted and sluggish, even after a good night's sleep.

WHAT ARE SOME OTHER SIGNS THAT YOU MIGHT HAVE TYPE 2 DIABETES?

If you have type 2 diabetes, you have a higher risk of suffering from various other health problems. Sometimes, it is these secondary issues that lead people to seek medical attention for their diabetes rather than the symptoms listed above.

For instance, nerve damage is one common complication that many people with Type 2 diabetes encounter. If you have high blood sugar levels for an extended period, your nerves can get damaged or even destroyed, leading to a condition called neuropathy. This can cause you to feel numbness, tingling, or loss of sensation in your limbs.

People with diabetes can also develop a condition known as autonomic neuropathy. This happens when the nerves controlling the heart and blood vessels get damaged or destroyed. Consequently, it may be harder to control your blood pressure, heartbeat, and digestion.

High blood sugar levels damage the blood vessels and lead to inflammation in the kidneys, which can eventually cause kidney disease. People with Type 2 diabetes are also 2-4 times more likely to develop eye-related complications than those without it.

Moreover, people with diabetes may also experience sleep apnea, a condition characterized by the cessation of breathing for short periods during sleep. Obesity is the primary contributing factor behind both Type 2 diabetes and sleep apnea.

Another less-known symptom of Type 2 diabetes is dementia. People with uncontrolled blood sugar levels are at a higher risk of developing Alzheimer's disease or other related disorders. In some studies, it has been found that poor control of blood sugar is linked to a more rapid decline in memory and other cognitive functions.

Finally, Type 2 diabetes can affect your skin in various ways. We may notice yellow, reddish, or brown patches on our skin, and around the eyes, they may occur in clusters that look like pimples. You may notice the appearance of velvety, dark areas on your skin. You may also experience skin infections, open sores, shin spots, red-yellow bumps, dryness, itchiness, and skin tags.

WHAT IS THE DIFFERENCE BETWEEN TYPE 1 AND TYPE 2 DIABETES?

These two types of diabetes are commonly grouped together, but they are very different. In fact, they have a different impact on your health, diagnosis, and treatment.

So, what is the main difference between type 1 and type 2 diabetes? Type 1 diabetes is an autoimmune disease where your immune system attacks and destroys the cells in your pancreas that make insulin. Insulin is a hormone that allows your body to use sugar for energy.

Without insulin, sugar builds up in your bloodstream and can lead to serious health problems. Type 1 diabetes typically develops in childhood or young adulthood and requires lifelong insulin therapy.

On the other hand, type 2 diabetes is a metabolic disorder where your body either doesn't produce enough insulin or can't use insulin effectively. This is known as insulin resistance.

Unlike type 1 diabetes, type 2 diabetes can be prevented or delayed with lifestyle changes like a healthy diet and regular exercise. However, if left untreated, it can lead to serious health complications.

Type 1 diabetes affects only 8% of people with diabetes, while type 2 diabetes accounts for about 90% of cases, as I mentioned earlier. However, the signs and symptoms of both types of diabetes can be similar, such as increased thirst, frequent urination, and blurred vision.

Another difference between type 1 and type 2 diabetes is related to the risk factors. Type 1 diabetes is thought to be caused by a combination of genetic and environmental factors, such as exposure to viruses and other triggers.

Type 2 diabetes, on the other hand, is associated with risk factors like obesity, inactivity, and unhealthy eating habits. If you have a family history of diabetes, you are also at higher risk of developing type 2 diabetes.

Diagnosing the two different types of diabetes is also different - something I'll address in greater detail below.

HOW IS DIABETES DIAGNOSED?

The most common way of diagnosing type 2 diabetes is through the A1C test. This test measures your average blood sugar level over the past two to three months.

If your A1C test results indicate a value of 6.5% or higher on two separate tests, then you have diabetes. However, if you are experiencing certain conditions or if the A1C test is not available, your healthcare provider may use the following tests to diagnose diabetes.

There is also a random blood sugar test where blood sugar values are expressed in milligrams of sugar per deciliter of blood. Regardless of when you last ate, a blood sugar level of 200 mg/dL or higher indicates diabetes if you are also experiencing symptoms like frequent urination and extreme thirst.

Another test that your healthcare provider may use to diagnose diabetes is a fasting blood sugar test. Your healthcare provider takes a blood sample after you have not eaten overnight.

If your fasting blood glucose level measures less than 100 mg/dL, it is considered healthy. If your level is between 100-125 mg/dL, it is diagnosed as prediabetes.

However, if it is 126 mg/dL or higher on two separate tests, you likely have diabetes.

For the oral glucose tolerance test, you'll need to not eat for a certain amount of time and then drink a sugary liquid at your healthcare provider's office. Your glucose level is then tested periodically for two hours. This test is less commonly used than the others, except during pregnancy.

Now that you know the basics about type 2 diabetes, including its symptoms and diagnosis, let's talk a bit more about blood sugar and insulin. After all, these are two of the most important factors to consider (and insulin, the most important element in the treatment of diabetes) when you're coming up with a treatment plan.

Grab a glass of water and a snack, then come back and keep reading. I'll be here waiting for you!

2

UNDERSTANDING INSULIN AND BLOOD SUGAR

"Insulin is not a cure for diabetes; it is a treatment. It enables the diabetic to burn sufficient carbohydrates so that proteins and fats may be added to the diet in sufficient quantities to provide energy for the economic burdens of life."

— FREDERICK BANTING

If you're someone who's struggling with diabetes, chances are you've heard the word 'insulin' thrown around a lot. But what's insulin, and why is it so important when it comes to diabetes management?

When you eat, your digestive system breaks down the food into glucose, which gets absorbed into your bloodstream. However, for glucose to enter your cells and provide energy, it needs insulin. Insulin is a hormone produced by the pancreas that helps regulate blood sugar levels in your body. If you're diabetic, there are problems with this - the body has become resistant to insulin and can't use it effectively.

Let's take a closer look at how insulin and glucose work together.

WHAT ROLE DOES INSULIN PLAY IN THE BODY?

If you're living with diabetes, you've probably heard the word "insulin" more often than you'd like. This hormone, produced by the pancreas, plays a crucial role in regulating your blood sugar levels.

But how?

Insulin is a hormone that helps our bodies convert glucose (a type of sugar) into energy. When we eat carbohydrates, our digestive system breaks them down into glucose, which then enters the bloodstream. This signals the pancreas to release insulin, which acts like a key to unlock the cells in our muscles, liver, and fat tissue, allowing them to absorb glucose from the blood and use it for energy.

Without insulin, our cells would be starved of glucose, and our blood sugar levels would skyrocket, leading to a condition called hyperglycemia. Over time, uncontrolled hyperglycemia can damage our nerves, blood vessels, kidneys, and eyes, causing serious complications like heart disease, blindness, and nerve damage.

For people living with type 1 diabetes, their pancreas cannot produce insulin, so they must take insulin injections or use an insulin pump to regulate their blood sugar levels. For those with type 2 diabetes, their body becomes resistant to the effects of insulin, so they may need to take medication to help their body use insulin more effectively.

Aside from its role in regulating blood sugar, insulin also plays several other important functions in the body. For example, it helps to stimulate the growth and repair of cells, promotes the storage of fat, and inhibits the breakdown of stored glucose and fat. In addition, insulin acts as a signal to the kidneys to reabsorb glucose, aiding in its conservation.

Interestingly, insulin can also affect our hunger and satiety levels. When we eat a meal, our blood sugar levels spike, causing insulin to be released and helping our cells absorb glucose.

But this also causes a drop in our blood sugar levels, which signals the brain to feel hungry and crave more food. However, insulin also triggers the release of hormones that make us feel full, so we don't overeat.

WHAT IS BLOOD GLUCOSE?

Simply put, blood glucose is the sugar that's carried in our blood and provides energy to our cells. It comes from the food we eat and is one of the main things our bodies use for fuel. Sounds important, right?

But for diabetics, keeping blood glucose levels within a healthy range can be a challenge. In type 1 diabetes, the pancreas can't produce insulin, a hormone that helps regulate blood glucose levels. In type 2 diabetes, the body doesn't use insulin as effectively as it should. Both types can lead to high blood glucose levels, which can cause a variety of health complications if left uncontrolled.

So why is it so important to keep blood glucose levels in check? First and foremost, it can help prevent long-term complications like nerve damage, kidney damage, and eye damage. But it can also have an immediate impact on how we feel day-to-day. High blood glucose levels can make us feel tired, thirsty, and generally unwell. On the other hand, low blood glucose levels can lead to shakiness, dizziness, and even unconsciousness.

Managing blood glucose levels as a diabetic can be a full-time job, but there are a variety of tools and strategies that can make it easier. One of the most important is monitoring your levels regularly through blood glucose testing. You may need to do this several times a day, depending on your treatment plan and the advice of your healthcare provider.

Again, I'll have more information on this for you later in this book.

WHAT ROLE DOES THE PANCREAS PLAY?

As a diabetic, you are probably aware that insulin and glucose management are vital to your health. Both factors play a crucial role in keeping your body functioning correctly. However, do you know which organ in your body is responsible for regulating insulin and glucose levels?

Truth be told, the pancreas is somewhat of an unsung hero when it comes to glucose and insulin management.

The pancreas is a small, spongy gland that is located behind your stomach. It is responsible for the secretion of two important hormones, insulin and glucagon, which regulate blood glucose levels in the body. Insulin is produced by beta cells in the pancreas, which plays a critical role in allowing glucose to enter cells and produce energy.

Meanwhile, glucagon is released by alpha cells in the pancreas and raises blood glucose levels when it drops too low.

Most people are familiar with insulin and know that it's essential for managing blood glucose levels. After we eat, our pancreas releases insulin into our bloodstream, which helps cells absorb glucose from food. In a perfect world, our pancreas produces just enough insulin for our body's needs.

Unfortunately, for diabetics, there's an imbalance - either too little insulin or too much. This imbalance can lead to hyperglycemia (high blood sugar) or hypoglycemia (low blood sugar) - both of which can have harmful effects on your body.

When your body is unable to produce enough insulin or becomes resistant to insulin, it can lead to diabetes.

HOW DOES GLUCOSE METABOLISM WORK?

Glucose, a simple sugar, serves as the primary source of fuel for our bodies. After consuming carbohydrates, such as bread and fruit, they are broken down into glucose molecules in the digestive system. This glucose then enters the bloodstream, where it is transported to cells throughout the body.

To enter these cells, glucose requires insulin, a hormone produced by the pancreas. Insulin attaches to the cells' receptors, signaling for them to open and absorb glucose from the bloodstream. Once inside the cells, glucose can be used for energy or stored for later use.

When the body doesn't produce enough insulin or is unable to properly use it, glucose cannot enter the cells efficiently. As a result, glucose builds up in the bloodstream, leading to high blood sugar levels - diabetes.

Beyond diabetes, glucose metabolism also plays a role in other areas of health. For instance, high blood sugar levels can lead to inflammation, which has been linked to a host of health issues, such as heart disease and cancer. Understanding and managing glucose metabolism can help minimize these risks.

WHAT MAKES YOUR GLUCOSE METABOLISM GET OUT OF WHACK?

If you're a diabetic, then you know how finicky your glucose metabolism can be. One minute it's cruising along, and the next, it's as if it's been thrown off its rocker. But what exactly makes this happen? You won't be surprised to hear that many of the factors that cause an imbalance in your glucose metabolism are the same ones discussed as risk factors for diabetes earlier in this book, in the last chapter.

The most obvious culprit behind a dysfunctional glucose metabolism is a poor diet. Unhealthy eating habits, such as consuming excessive amounts of refined sugars, can lead to spikes in blood sugar, which may cause your body to overload on insulin. In turn, this can cause insulin resistance, which impairs your body's ability to control blood sugar levels effectively.

Regular exercise is essential in maintaining optimal glucose metabolism. Exercise increases your insulin sensitivity, allowing your body to use insulin more effectively.

Studies have also shown that physical activity can decrease insulin resistance, which improves glucose tolerance in people with diabetes. A lack of exercise, therefore, can exacerbate glucose metabolism issues and may lead to complications in the long run.

Did you know that your genes may hold the key to your glucose metabolism, too? Research has shown that certain genes can increase the likelihood of developing insulin resistance, leading to high blood sugar levels over time. Having a family history of diabetes puts you at a higher risk of developing glucose metabolism issues, and it's something that you should keep in mind when managing your condition.

Chronic stress is another important factor that can wreak havoc on your glucose metabolism. When your body is under stress, it releases stress hormones such as cortisol and adrenaline, which can cause an increase in blood sugar levels. Over time, chronic stress can impair your body's response to insulin and may lead to insulin resistance, which affects your glucose metabolism.

Finally, certain medications can also affect your glucose metabolism. Drugs such as corticosteroids (pain and inflammation), diuretics (water pill), and beta-blockers (heart and blood pressure) have all been known to cause glucose metabolism issues, either by increasing insulin resistance or by impairing your body's ability to produce insulin.

So, if you're taking any medications that may be affecting your blood sugar levels, it's crucial to talk to your doctor about possible alternatives or adjustments.

CARBS AND DIABETES

When you have diabetes, controlling your blood sugar levels is essential to maintaining your overall health. One of the critical considerations is how many carbohydrates you consume every day. Carbohydrates (carbs) are broken down into sugar in the body.

Despite the many myths about carbs and diabetes, they're not enemies! In fact, they are essential for providing energy to your body and keeping it running smoothly. But just like with every food, it's essential to calculate your carb intake and choose the right type of carbs.

Let's take a closer look.

What Are Carbs?

Macronutrients include protein, fats, and carbs; these are the main sources of fuel that allow your body to function. Carbohydrates provide glucose, which is the primary energy source for your body. Carbohydrates are found in many foods, including grains, fruits, vegetables, and beans.

When you eat carbs, your body converts them into glucose, which your cells use for energy. It's essential to maintain an adequate supply of carbs and control your blood glucose levels at the same time.

How Do Carbs Fit Into a Healthy Diet?

Carbs are an essential part of a healthy diet, but it's crucial to choose the right type of carbs, such as whole grains, fruits, vegetables, and beans, rather than refined carbs like pastries, candies, and white bread.

Now, that's not to say that you must ban bread entirely. You just need to set limits. Scot Lester, who was diagnosed with diabetes in 2012, found that he was able to continue eating carbohydrates as long as he limited himself to just 35 grams per day (a challenge, still, since he was a self-described sweet tooth).

Roger Hare is another example. When he wants to splurge, he tests his blood sugar levels first. If they're lower, he allows himself a bit more carbs - if not, he limits it. This helps him stay in tune with what his body needs.

You should aim to include carbohydrates in every meal or snack, but don't overdo it. One way to calculate your daily carb intake is by talking to your healthcare professional or even better, a nutritionist. They will help you determine the number of carbs you should consume daily based on your age, weight, and other factors.

Types of Carbohydrates

Let's break down carbs even more! There are three types of carbohydrates: sugars, starches, and fiber.

Sugars are the simplest type of carb, found in many foods such as fruits, syrups, and honey. Starches are a complex type of carb that the body breaks down into glucose, found in grains, potatoes, and legumes.

The third type of carb is fiber, which is not digested by the body, found in vegetables, whole grains, and fruits. To maintain healthy blood sugar levels, choose unrefined and complex carbs whenever you can. Refined carbs are processed whereas unrefined contain more natural fiber.

Whole and unprocessed carbs (unrefined and complex) include whole grains, beans, fruits, and vegetables. These are all great sources of fiber, vitamins, minerals, and phytonutrients.

Simple and processed carbs (refined and simple) include sugar and processed grains that have been stripped of all bran, fiber, and nutrients such as white bread, white flour, pizza dough, pasta, pastries, desserts, white rice and often breakfast cereals.

Net Carbs and Glycemic Index

The concept of net carbs was introduced to help people with diabetes manage their carb intake. Net carbs are the total number of carbohydrates in a food minus the fiber content that the body doesn't digest. A food that has a lot of carbohydrates but also has a lot of fiber will have fewer net carbs than one that has the same amount of carbohydrates, but less fiber.

The glycemic index (GI) is another term used for carbohydrates. It's a scale that measures how quickly a particular food raises blood sugar levels.

Foods with a high glycemic index rank high on the scale, and those with a low glycemic index rank low. Foods with a lower glycemic index are usually better for people with diabetes since they don't cause a sudden spike in blood sugar levels.

High glycemic index foods include white bread, white rice, breakfast cereals and cereal bars, cakes, cookies, potatoes, fries, chips, some fruits such as watermelon and pineapple, and sweetened yogurt.

Low glycemic index foods include green vegetables, most fruits, raw carrots, kidney beans, chickpeas, and lentils.

Don't get too caught up in the terminology, this is just to give you an idea in case your medical provider or nutritionist mentions these terms.

How Many Carbs Do You Need?

The number of carbohydrates you need varies based on your age, weight, gender, and activity level.

Most people require an intake of at least 130 grams a day. A pro marathon runner might eat more than 500 grams of carbohydrates, while someone who is inactive might need as little as 50.

However, when you have diabetes, you would need to regulate your intake of carbs due to its impact on blood sugar levels. That's why you will want to consult with your dietitian or diabetes educator to help you determine the right amount of carbs per day for you.

Carbohydrates and Your Health

Raise your hand if you have ever been at a restaurant and stare blankly at the menu, trying to figure out which dish has the least amount of carbs. Or you've experienced that dreaded feeling when you prick your finger to check your blood sugar, only to see the numbers jump after consuming a high-carb meal.

As a diabetic, you need to be cautious of the amount and type of carbs we consume because our bodies do not produce enough insulin or can't use it properly to regulate our blood sugar levels.

It is important to remember that everyone's body processes carbs differently. What might cause a spike in your blood sugar might not have the same effect on someone else. Keep track of the foods you eat and monitor your blood sugar levels to see how certain foods affect you personally.

Choosing Your Carbohydrates Wisely

Now, when it comes to choosing your carbs wisely, there are a few things to keep in mind. First, aim for complex carbohydrates instead of simple carbohydrates.

Complex carbs, again, take longer to digest, providing a slower release of glucose into the bloodstream, which helps prevent blood sugar spikes. Good sources of complex carbs include sweet potatoes, brown rice, quinoa, and legumes. On the other hand, simple carbs such as candy, soda, and white bread are quickly broken down into glucose, causing a rapid rise in blood sugar levels.

Another crucial factor to consider is portion size. While it is important to be mindful of the type of carbs you're consuming, the amount you eat can also impact your blood sugar levels. Try to stick to recommended serving sizes for foods that contain carbs and be mindful of portion sizes when dining out.

Remember that not all carbs are equal. Foods with a high GI (glycemic index) score (such as white bread and sugary drinks) cause a rapid spike in blood sugar, whole foods with a low GI score (such as most fruits and vegetables) have a slower effect on blood sugar levels. Aim for foods with a lower GI score to help keep your blood sugar levels steady.

HOW INSULIN RESISTANCE OCCURS

Insulin resistance is a condition that impairs your body's ability to use insulin, a hormone that helps regulate blood sugar levels. It's a common problem among people with type 2 diabetes, but it can also affect those with type 1 diabetes and other health conditions as well.

To understand insulin resistance, let's quickly recap how insulin works in the body. Insulin is produced by the pancreas and helps your body use glucose (sugar) from the food you eat for energy.

When you eat, your body releases insulin to help move glucose from your bloodstream into your cells. Think of insulin as a key that unlocks the door to your cells, allowing glucose to enter.

However, if you have insulin resistance, your cells become resistant to the effects of insulin. This means that your body needs to produce more insulin to get the same amount of glucose into your cells. Over time, this can lead to high insulin levels in the bloodstream, which can cause a range of health problems, including type 2 diabetes, heart disease, and obesity.

There are several factors that can contribute to insulin resistance, including genetics, lifestyle, and body weight. For example, if you have a family history of diabetes or are overweight, you may be more likely to develop insulin resistance.

Similarly, a sedentary lifestyle and a diet high in processed and sugary foods can also increase your risk.

Fortunately, there are several steps you can take to manage insulin resistance and improve your overall health.

One of the most effective strategies is to make lifestyle changes, such as exercising regularly and eating a healthy diet that's low in sugar and refined carbohydrates. This can help your body become more sensitive to insulin, reducing the need for high insulin levels.

I'll give you more tips later in this book but know that medication can also be prescribed to help manage insulin resistance. These medications work by increasing insulin sensitivity or reducing insulin resistance in the body. They are usually prescribed in combination with lifestyle changes and can be very effective in controlling blood sugar levels and preventing diabetes complications.

THE IMPACT OF HIGH BLOOD SUGAR ON THE BODY

Sugar is in everything we eat, from cakes and sweets to our everyday food choices, like bread and pasta. However, when enjoying sugar in copious quantities, it can become deadly for diabetics.

High blood sugar, or hyperglycemia, occurs when your body cannot produce or use insulin correctly. Again, insulin is responsible for maintaining your blood sugar levels. If left untreated, high blood sugar can cause damage to your body's vital organs, such as your heart, kidneys, and eyes. And it can cause neurological problems like numbness and tingling in the extremities.

Moderate to severe cases of high blood sugar can lead to a condition called diabetic ketoacidosis. This happens when your body starts breaking down fat for energy instead of glucose and leads to the production of ketones.

Ketones are like acids that accumulate in the blood. They can cause severe damage to your blood vessels and lead to low blood pressure, a rapid heartbeat, and even coma.

While high blood sugar can go unnoticed in its initial stages, some telltale signs include fatigue, dry mouth, increased thirst, frequent urination, and headaches. Other symptoms include blurred vision, nerve damage, loss of consciousness, and even heart attack.

To manage high blood sugar levels, you need to commit to a healthy lifestyle. It includes a healthy diet, regular exercise, and taking any prescribed medication. To keep your blood sugar in check, you will need to control your carbohydrate intake, stay hydrated, and monitor your glucose levels regularly. Taking medication as prescribed and adjusting it according to your doctor's recommendations can help control your blood sugar levels.

It can be challenging to manage high blood sugar levels without support. That is why having a good support system is essential. You can seek support from diabetes support groups, family, friends, and even healthcare professionals.

Together, you can manage your blood sugar levels and avoid complications - and remember, you have a built-in community right here in this book, so stick with me as we go through some lifestyle modifications you can easily make.

THE RELATIONSHIP BETWEEN INSULIN AND BLOOD SUGAR

Again, insulin is a hormone that's produced in the pancreas, a gland located just behind your stomach. Its primary function is to regulate the amount of glucose (sugar) in your bloodstream.

When you eat carbohydrates, your body breaks them down into glucose molecules, which are then transported to your cells by the bloodstream. Insulin allows glucose to enter and be used as energy. Without insulin, glucose would accumulate in your bloodstream, leading to a condition known as hyperglycemia or high blood sugar.

However, in some cases, the body's production of insulin is impaired, leading to the condition we know all too well as diabetes. In type 1 diabetes, the pancreas doesn't produce enough insulin, while in type 2 diabetes, the body becomes resistant to insulin, leading to a buildup of glucose in the bloodstream.

To manage diabetes, diabetics may need to inject synthetic insulin or take medications that enhance the body's response to insulin.

While insulin is essential for regulating blood sugar, too much of it can also be harmful. When you eat a large meal or consume too many carbohydrates, your body releases a surge of insulin to deal with the excess glucose. This can cause your blood sugar levels to drop rapidly, leading to a condition known as hypoglycemia or low blood sugar.

Symptoms of hypoglycemia include dizziness, confusion, sweating, and even loss of consciousness in severe cases. To avoid hypoglycemia, diabetics may need to monitor their blood sugar levels frequently and adjust their medication or food intake accordingly.

The relationship between insulin and blood sugar is dynamic and complex, with many factors influencing their interaction.

For diabetics, understanding how insulin affects their blood sugar levels is crucial to managing their condition. Whether you're newly diagnosed or have been living with diabetes for years, it's never too late to educate yourself about your body's inner workings. Hopefully, this chapter has helped you to do just that!

Now that you know what glucose and insulin are, you hopefully have a better understanding of how your body works - and what can go wrong.

In the next chapter, we'll explore the root causes of diabetes and how these root causes can exacerbate the problem if they aren't properly managed. It might be overwhelming, but knowing about all the different variables that are at play can make a huge difference in managing your symptoms.

Ready to get started? Keep reading to learn more...

3

THE CAUSES AND PREVENTION OF DIABETES

"Diabetes sounds like you're going to die when you hear it. I was immediately frightened. But once I got a better idea of what it was and that it was something I could manage myself, I was comforted."

— NICK JONAS

Diabetes. It's a word that can leave people feeling frightened and helpless. It can seem like a death sentence, but it's important to remember that people with diabetes can still lead long, healthy lives.

The key is understanding the causes of diabetes and taking steps to prevent them from derailing you.

Now that you know what diabetes is, we need to take a closer look at some of the causes. While the exact causes of both Type 1 and Type 2 diabetes are not fully understood, there are several factors that can increase your risk, especially when they exist together.

Let's take a closer look.

WHAT GENETIC FACTORS CONTRIBUTE TO DIABETES?

One of the strongest predictors of type 2 diabetes is having a family history of the disease. If a close relative, such as a parent or sibling, has the condition, your risk of developing it increases. This is because type 2 diabetes has a significant genetic component.

Scientists have identified several genes that are associated with type 2 diabetes risk, including TCF7L2, CDKAL1, HHEX, and FTO. These genes are involved in regulating insulin production and glucose metabolism, and variations in their DNA sequences can lead to impaired insulin secretion and increased insulin resistance.

Another important factor that affects type 2 diabetes risk is ethnicity. Certain ethnic groups, such as African Americans, Hispanics, Native Americans, and Asian Americans, are more likely to develop the condition than others.

This is partly due to genetic differences that affect insulin sensitivity and glucose metabolism. For example, African Americans and Hispanics tend to have a higher prevalence of the TCF7L2 gene variant, which is associated with a higher risk of type 2 diabetes.

By contrast, Native Americans have a higher prevalence of genetic variants that affect lipid metabolism (cholesterol), which can increase their risk of developing diabetes.

Obesity is a major risk factor for type 2 diabetes, and genetics can also play a role in this relationship. Researchers have identified certain genetic variants that are associated with higher body mass index (BMI) and increased adiposity (fat mass).

These variants can affect the regulation of appetite, energy expenditure, and lipid metabolism, all of which can contribute to the development of obesity and type 2 diabetes. Some of the genes that have been implicated in this process include FTO, MC4R, and PPARG.

In addition to DNA sequences, epigenetic modifications also play a role in the development of type 2 diabetes. Epigenetics refers to changes in gene expression that do not involve alterations to the DNA sequence itself. Nutrition and food sources have an impact on epigenetics (gene expression).

Factors such as diet, exercise, and environmental toxins can all influence epigenetic modifications and affect the risk of diabetes. For example, studies have shown that maternal exposure to a high-fat diet during pregnancy can alter the epigenetic marks on the offspring's DNA, leading to increased diabetes risk later in life.

Finally, it is important to recognize that the relationship between genetics and type 2 diabetes is complex and multifaceted. In many cases, genetic factors may only increase the risk of diabetes under certain environmental conditions.

For example, individuals with a high genetic risk of diabetes may only develop the disease if they also lead a sedentary lifestyle or consume a diet high in sugar and fat. By contrast, those with a low genetic risk may still develop diabetes if they are exposed to certain environmental risk factors.

WHICH LIFESTYLE CHOICES IMPACT DIABETES RISK?

Let's focus on the lifestyle choices that can impact diabetes risk and what you can do to decrease your risk.

Food

The food you eat plays a big role in your risk of developing diabetes. Eating a diet that is high in sugar, refined carbohydrates, and unhealthy fats can all contribute to an increased risk of diabetes.

On the other hand, a diet that is rich in fruits, vegetables, whole grains, and lean protein can help lower your risk. Be mindful of your food choices by reading nutrition labels and aiming for a balanced diet.

Exercise

Regular exercise is also important when it comes to reducing your risk of diabetes. Exercise helps to improve insulin sensitivity, which means your cells are better able to use insulin to process glucose. This can help to keep blood sugar levels within a healthy range.

Even just 30 minutes of physical activity per day can make a big difference in reducing your risk of diabetes. The recommended minimum goal is 150 minutes per week.

Medication

If you already have diabetes, it's important to take your medication as prescribed by your healthcare provider. This can help to keep your blood sugar levels under control and reduce your risk of complications.

Make sure to talk to your healthcare provider if you have any concerns about taking your medication.

Illness

Certain illnesses, such as high blood pressure, heart disease, and obesity, can increase your risk of diabetes. By managing any existing health conditions, you have, you can reduce your risk of developing diabetes. This includes maintaining a healthy weight, eating a balanced diet, and exercising regularly.

Alcohol

Drinking alcohol in moderation is okay, but not recommended, for people with diabetes. However, excessive drinking can increase your risk of developing diabetes - so it should be avoided. If you choose to drink alcohol, do so in moderation and make sure to eat food with your drink.

Menstruation and Menopause

For women, hormonal changes during menstruation and menopause can affect blood sugar levels. It's important for women with diabetes to stay on top of these changes and work with their healthcare provider to manage their diabetes. This may involve adjusting medication doses or monitoring blood sugar levels more closely during these times.

OTHER RISK FACTORS FOR DIABETES

Although the factors listed above are some of the most often-cited reasons for why people develop type 2 diabetes, they certainly aren't the only ones. Here are a few more.

Obesity

As mentioned, being overweight is a well-known risk factor for type 2 diabetes.

However, it's not just about the total number of pounds a person carries, but also about where that weight is distributed.

Carrying extra weight in the midsection or having a high waist-to-hip ratio, increases the risk of developing diabetes. This is because abdominal fat produces chemicals that can interfere with the body's ability to produce insulin, the hormone responsible for regulating blood sugar levels.

If you have a large waist circumference, losing even a small amount of weight can help improve your blood sugar control.

Age

As we get older, the risk of developing diabetes increases. This is partly due to lifestyle factors, such as decreased physical activity, poorer dietary choices, and weight gain. However, there may also be genetic factors at play.

The incidence of diabetes increases significantly after age 45, with most cases occurring in those over 65. If you fall into this age range, it's important to be vigilant about monitoring your blood sugar levels and adhering to a healthy lifestyle to help prevent or manage diabetes.

Sedentary Lifestyle

Leading a sedentary lifestyle, characterized by little to no physical activity, is another risk factor for diabetes. Exercise helps the body use insulin more efficiently, which in turn helps to regulate blood sugar levels.

On the other hand, a lack of exercise can cause insulin resistance, which makes it harder for the body to use insulin effectively. This risk factor is especially relevant for those who have a family history of diabetes or other related conditions. If you're not currently active, talk to your doctor about how to start a safe and effective exercise regimen.

Family History

If you have a family member with diabetes, your own risk of developing the condition is higher.

However, it's important to note that family history is just one of many risk factors and does not automatically guarantee a diabetes diagnosis.

Still, having a close relative with diabetes (especially a parent or sibling) can make it more important to manage other risk factors, such as weight, blood pressure, and cholesterol levels. It's also important to stay on top of regular diabetes screenings and to be aware of any early symptoms that may arise.

THE ROLE OF SLEEP AND STRESS IN DIABETES PREVENTION

Diet and exercise are typical measures used to manage the condition. However, what most people don't realize is that sleep and stress play a crucial role in diabetes prevention as well.

Lack of sleep or poor-quality sleep can contribute to the development of type 2 diabetes in several ways. For starters, it can lead to insulin resistance and an increased risk of type 2 diabetes.

Studies have shown that people who sleep less than six hours per night have a higher risk of developing type 2 diabetes than those who sleep more. Also, poor sleep can affect our stress hormone levels, leading to insulin resistance, inflammation, and obesity.

Chronic stress can increase your risk of developing diabetes. This is because stress hormones can cause an increase in blood sugar levels. To manage stress, try activities such as yoga, meditation, or deep breathing exercises. Stress levels can have a direct impact on your blood sugar levels. Chronic stress can lead to insulin resistance, which could ultimately result in type 2 diabetes. Cortisol, the stress hormone, raises blood sugar levels, making it difficult to manage the condition.

STEROID USE AND DIABETES

If you've used steroids or are currently using steroids, you might be curious about how they will come into play in terms of managing your diabetes.

What Are Steroids?

Steroids are synthetic substances that are designed to mimic the effects of the hormone testosterone.

They are commonly used in medicine to treat hormonal issues, muscle loss, and to trigger muscle growth. Steroids can be taken orally, injected, or applied topically to the skin. They also come in different forms, such as creams, gels, and sprays.

The two main types of steroids are corticosteroids and anabolic steroids. Corticosteroids are typically used for treating inflammation or autoimmune diseases, such as asthma and lupus.

They work by reducing inflammation in the body and, in turn, easing symptoms. Anabolic steroids, on the other hand, are used to build muscle mass and strength, which is often the reason why people who work out use them.

How Steroids Impact Blood Glucose Levels

Steroids are known to increase blood glucose levels as they affect the way your body metabolizes sugar.

Normally, the body produces insulin to help regulate blood sugar levels. However, when you take steroids, this can lead to insulin resistance, which can cause elevated blood sugars. Steroids can also cause the liver to release stored glucose into the bloodstream, further increasing blood glucose levels.

If you're taking steroids and notice an increase in your blood glucose levels, it's essential to speak with your doctor. They may recommend taking extra insulin or other medications to help regulate your blood sugars.

It's also important to note that not all steroids are equal when it comes to their impact on blood glucose levels. Some steroids, such as dexamethasone, have more significant impacts on blood glucose levels than others. Again, it's essential to speak with your doctor about the steroid you're taking and what you can do to help manage blood glucose level changes.

Diabetes Management When You Must Use Steroids

Steroids can affect glucose levels and insulin sensitivity, which is why it's essential to keep an eye on your diabetes management when taking them.

Check Glucose Levels More Often

Steroids can affect glucose levels, so it's essential to monitor them more frequently than usual. Frequent testing will help you catch any potential issues before they become a problem. If you find that your glucose levels are consistently higher than normal, speak to your healthcare team about adjusting your insulin dosage or medication.

Increase Insulin or Medication Dosage Based on Doctor Recommendations

If you're taking insulin or other diabetes medications, it may be necessary to adjust your dosage when taking steroids. Talk to your healthcare provider about increasing your insulin or medication dosage, as they may advise you to take more.

Don't take it upon yourself to adjust your insulin dosage without consulting your healthcare team, as it can lead to serious complications.

Monitor Urine and Blood Ketones

When taking steroids, your body may start producing ketones, which can be dangerous if left unchecked. Ketones are commonly found in individuals with type 1 diabetes, but individuals with type 2 diabetes can also develop them if their glucose levels are consistently high.

Monitoring your urine and blood ketones is crucial when taking steroids. Speak to your healthcare team about how to do this effectively, and what you should do if your levels become too high.

Now that you know some of the underlying causes of diabetes, it is time to move on - you know what the problem is, so how do you deal with it?

In the next few chapters, we will give you an overview of some of the options that are available to help you treat and manage your diabetes. We will start first with the broad options before we establish more specific steps you can take.

4

TREATMENT OPTIONS FOR DIABETES

"Think about it: heart disease and diabetes account for more deaths in the U.S. and worldwide than everything else combined. They are completely preventable through lifestyle habits without drugs or surgery."

— DEAN ORNISH

Being diagnosed with diabetes can be overwhelming, especially when it comes to figuring out the best treatment options available. Luckily, the medical community has made incredible strides in recent years, offering a plethora of ways to control and manage this chronic illness.

Insulin is great. With over a hundred years of use, insulin is one of the most reliable and effective treatment options for diabetes.

However, it's certainly not the only option. With the right treatment plan and medical guidance, diabetes doesn't have to hold you back from living your best life.

Here are some of the other treatment options for diabetes so that you have plenty of information at your disposal when you meet with your doctor.

LIFESTYLE CHANGES AS A FIRST-LINE TREATMENT

The good news is that there are many things you can do to manage your type 2 diabetes - without medication. While there is no substitution for the right medication when you truly need it, that medication will be significantly more effective if you combine it with certain lifestyle adjustments.

A patient from Johns Hopkins who was diagnosed with diabetes at age 50 says "It's a lifestyle change – it impacts every part of your life (medications, meals, etc.). If you can realize this earlier on, you'll get under control much more quickly."

One of the most important lifestyle changes you can make when you have diabetes is to eat a healthy, balanced diet. This means avoiding sugary and processed foods and opting for lean proteins, whole grains, and plenty of fruits and vegetables.

Exercise is another important lifestyle change that can help manage diabetes. Regular physical activity can improve insulin sensitivity, which can help lower your blood sugar levels.

Maintaining a healthy weight is important for people with diabetes because excess body fat can make it more difficult for the body to use insulin effectively. Losing just a few pounds can improve insulin sensitivity and help lower your blood sugar levels.

Stress can cause a rise in blood sugar levels, making it important to find ways to manage stress effectively. Whether it's through meditation, deep breathing, or spending time with friends and family, finding ways to reduce stress can help improve your overall wellbeing and help manage diabetes.

And finally, it's important to monitor your blood sugar levels regularly to make sure they're within a healthy range. Your doctor can advise you on how often you should check your blood sugar levels and what your target range should be.

MEDICATION FOR BLOOD SUGAR CONTROL

Apart from making necessary changes in diet and exercise, medication plays a significant role in keeping blood sugar levels in check. With a wide range of medications available in the market, it can be quite daunting to choose which best suits your needs.

Here are some of the most common options that might be prescribed.

Metformin

Metformin is one of the most prescribed medications for blood sugar control. It works by reducing glucose production in the liver and enhancing insulin sensitivity. The advantages of metformin include reduced risk of hypoglycemia, improved cholesterol levels, and modest weight loss. The disadvantage of metformin is that it can cause digestive side effects such as nausea, vomiting, diarrhea, and stomach cramps. Metformin also depletes vitamin B12 which often requires supplementation.

Sulfonylureas

Sulfonylureas are oral medications that stimulate the pancreas to produce and release more insulin. They are generally inexpensive and effective in lowering blood sugar levels. Sulfonylureas are associated with an increased risk of hypoglycemia, weight gain, and cardiovascular side effects in some people. Examples include glipizide, glyburide, and glimepiride.

Thiazolidinediones (TZDs)

TZDs are oral medications that improve insulin sensitivity and reduce glucose production in the liver. They are typically used in conjunction with other medications and can cause fluid retention, weight gain, and an increased risk of heart failure. Examples include rosiglitazone and pioglitazone.

Dipeptidyl peptidase-4 inhibitors (DPP-4 inhibitors)

DPP-4 inhibitors are oral medications that help lower blood sugar levels by preventing the breakdown of a hormone called glucagon-like peptide-1 (GLP-1).

The advantages of DPP-4 inhibitors include a lower risk of hypoglycemia, weight neutrality, and a lower risk of cardiovascular side effects. They can cause upper respiratory tract infections, headaches, and gastrointestinal side effects.

These medications are often expensive because generics are not available. These include Januvia (sitagliptin), Onglyza (saxagliptin), Tradjenta (linagliptin), and Nesina (alogliptin).

GLP-1 receptor agonists

GLP-1 receptor agonists are injectable medications that mimic the effects of GLP-1 and help lower blood sugar levels. They also reduce appetite, promote weight loss, and have a lower risk of hypoglycemia.

The disadvantage of GLP-1 receptor agonists is that they are expensive, require injections, and can cause gastrointestinal side effects such as nausea, vomiting, and diarrhea.

These medications are often expensive because generics are not available. These include Trulicity (dulaglutide), Bydureon (Exenatide) weekly, and Byetta (Exenatide) twice daily, Ozempic (semaglutide), Victoza (liraglutide), Wegovy (semaglutide) and Rybelsus (semaglutide). Rybelsus is the only drug in this class that is a tablet taken by mouth.

SGLT2 Inhibitors

SGLT2 inhibitors are another newer type of medication that work by blocking the reabsorption of glucose in the kidneys and increasing its excretion in the urine. This results in lower blood sugar levels and weight loss.

SGLT2 inhibitors have a low risk of hypoglycemia but can cause genital infections and increase the risk of dehydration and kidney problems.

Meglitinides

Meglitinides are a type of oral medication used to control blood sugar levels in people with type 2 diabetes. They work by stimulating the pancreas to secrete more insulin, which helps reduce blood sugar levels.

Meglitinides are often prescribed in combination with other diabetes medications such as Metformin and Insulin. Drugs in the Meglitinides class are usually taken before meals to help prevent high blood sugar spikes that typically occur after eating.

Meglitinides are beneficial to people who have undergone surgery, and those who can't control their blood sugar levels through lifestyle modifications alone. One major advantage of

Meglitinides over other diabetes medications is that they have a shorter duration of action. This means that they are processed more quickly by the body, and therefore have a lower risk of causing low blood sugar levels (hypoglycemia).

Mounjaro

Mounjaro is a new medication that combines two hormones called GIP and GLP-1. GIP stimulates insulin production in response to food, while GLP-1 helps to regulate blood sugar levels and decrease appetite.

This medication has shown promising results in clinical trials for people with type 2 diabetes, including improved blood sugar control and weight loss.

THE IMPORTANCE OF INSULIN THERAPY

One treatment option that has been known to bring incredible relief to people with type 2 diabetes is insulin therapy. Despite its obvious benefits, many people shy away from insulin therapy due to common myths and misconceptions surrounding its use.

Insulin therapy may be recommended as a standalone or in combination with other diabetes medications to achieve better glycemic control. The most common reason why people with type 2 diabetes decline insulin therapy is the misconception that it is only reserved for severe cases.

While insulin treatment may indeed be necessary for people with severe cases, insulin resistance can occur in anyone, regardless of symptom severity. In fact, starting insulin therapy earlier on in the illness can help achieve better glycemic control and improve long-term outcomes.

Another common myth about insulin therapy is the fear of needles. While it is understandable to feel anxious about self-injecting insulin, the reality is that needle technology has come a long way, and it is now easier and less painful to use insulin pens than it was before.

Furthermore, insulin injections are necessary for keeping blood sugar levels in check and can be an important aspect of diabetes management. Your medical practitioner will work with you to help you feel comfortable using the insulin pen and can suggest means of reducing discomfort during the injection process, such as numbing creams and adjusting injection sites.

Insulin therapy presents some unique benefits for people with type 2 diabetes, such as its ability to help regulate blood sugar levels dramatically. Insulin is created naturally by the pancreas and is used by your body to turn glucose into energy. In people with diabetes, however, the pancreas does not produce enough insulin or stops producing insulin altogether, causing blood glucose levels to soar. Insulin therapy can help compensate for the low or no insulin production demands of your body.

It is important to note that while insulin therapy is powerful, it should never replace a healthy diet and an active lifestyle. Combining insulin therapy with healthy lifestyle habits can lead to optimal results. Often lifestyle changes can result in decreasing medication requirements and enable your pancreas to regain function.

HOW, WHEN, AND WHY - MONITORING BLOOD SUGAR LEVELS

Monitoring blood sugar levels is extremely important for people who have type 2 diabetes.

It is a crucial aspect of diabetes control and can help prevent complications such as nerve damage, kidney disease, and blindness.

Let's take a closer look at how and why you should do this.

How and When to Test Your Blood Sugar

The first step to monitoring blood glucose levels is talking to your healthcare provider. They will recommend the frequency of testing based on your medical history and current diabetes management plan.

Some people with type 2 diabetes may need to test their blood sugar level multiple times a day, while others only need to do it once a week or as recommended by their doctor.

Daily Finger Sticks

The most common way to test blood glucose levels is through daily finger sticks. This involves pricking your finger with a small needle called a lancet and collecting a drop of blood onto a test strip.

The test strip is then inserted into a glucose meter, which will provide a reading of your blood glucose level. This is an affordable and straightforward method but can be quite painful due to frequent punctures.

Continuous Monitors

Advancements in technology have led to continuous glucose monitoring (CGM), which provides real-time glucose readings. A CGM device is inserted under the skin, and a sensor measures glucose levels in the fluid between cells. The readings are displayed on a monitor, providing a constant stream of information and a more comprehensive picture of blood glucose levels.

Further, some CGMs alert their users to changes in glucose levels when they are high, low, or fluctuating, assuring timely intervention from the health-care providers. Examples include Dexcom and Freestyle Libre.

However, CGM is relatively expensive and may not be covered by all insurance providers, while some people find the process of inserting and removing the device from their body uncomfortable.

What is Considered Normal Glucose?

First, a quick review about what glucose is. Glucose is a type of sugar that comes from the foods we eat. When glucose enters our blood, it's called blood glucose or blood sugar. It's the primary source of energy for our bodies, but too much of it can be harmful. That's why it's essential to keep our blood sugar levels within a healthy range.

What Numbers Should You See?

The normal glucose range is between 70-99 mg/dL when fasting. This means your blood was drawn after you haven't eaten for 8-12 hours.

What is Fasting and What Are Post Prandial Blood Sugar Levels?

Your blood sugar naturally rises after eating. How high it goes and how long it stays there depend on various factors, such as what you ate, how much you ate, and how fast your body digests food.

The normal postprandial blood sugar range is less than 140 mg/dL two hours after eating. However, the American Diabetes Association recommends keeping your postprandial levels under 180 mg/dL.

When Should You Be Concerned?

If your blood sugar levels are higher than the normal range, you could be at risk for complications such as kidney damage, nerve damage, blindness, heart disease, and stroke. But when should you be concerned?

The best piece of advice is to pay attention to your symptoms. If you feel thirsty, fatigued, have blurry vision, or experience frequent urination, that could indicate high blood sugar levels. You should also talk to your healthcare provider, who can help you understand your numbers and develop a plan to manage your blood sugar levels.

What is Hemoglobin A1C?

Hemoglobin A1C is a blood test that measures the amount of glucose (sugar) that has attached to hemoglobin, a protein in your red blood cells. The test gives you a picture of your average blood sugar levels over the past two to three months, rather than just at one moment in time.

That's important because blood sugar levels can fluctuate throughout the day, depending on what you eat, your physical activity, and other factors. By measuring your HbA1C, you and your healthcare team can get a better idea of how well your diabetes is being managed over time.

Normal Values and Goals

HbA1C levels are expressed as a percentage of the total hemoglobin in your blood. The higher the percentage, the higher your average blood glucose levels have been.

For people without diabetes, HbA1C levels are typically between 4 and 5.6%. However, people with type 2 diabetes may have higher levels of HbA1C due to the body's inability to use insulin effectively. The goal for most people with type 2 diabetes is to keep their HbA1C levels below 7%. However, your doctor may set a different target depending on your health status and other factors.

The American Diabetes Association advises people with diabetes to achieve an HbA1C level of 7% or lower, which translates to an average blood glucose level of 154 mg/dL. However, the target range may vary depending on your age, overall health status, and personal preferences.

If you're older or have underlying health concerns, your doctor may suggest a less stringent target range, like 8%. For pregnant women with diabetes, the goal range may also differ. Your healthcare provider will consider your unique circumstances to advise what target HbA1C level is best for you.

While the ADA has general guidelines on HbA1C goals, each patient's needs are unique. Your healthcare team, including your doctor, diabetes educator, and nutritionist, can help you set a customized target HbA1C level that aligns with your specific health status and preferences.

Generally, if you have a history of diabetes complications, your doctor may set a lower target HbA1C level. On the other hand, if you have underlying conditions that can cause hypoglycemia, your doctor may recommend a higher HbA1C range.

High levels of HbA1C over time can cause significant damage to your blood vessels, nerves, and organs. Along with other lifestyle changes and medications, monitoring your HbA1C levels regularly can help you stay on top of your diabetes management and live a healthier life.

Every 1% decrease in HbA1C results in a 40% reduction in the risk of developing diabetes-related complications. Therefore, achieving your target HbA1C goal is critical in preventing or delaying complications of diabetes.

Signs and Symptoms You Might Have Elevated Blood Sugar

When blood sugar levels get too high, it can lead to severe complications, and in some cases, it may lead to an emergency requiring immediate medical attention. Therefore, it's crucial to know the signs and symptoms of elevated blood sugar to act quickly and avoid any severe complications.

Here are some of the most common:

- **Extreme thirst**: You might feel excessively thirsty, and it can be challenging to quench your thirst even if you drink enough water. This symptom indicates that your body is trying to flush out excess sugar via urination, which leads to dehydration.
- **Frequent urination:** If you are urinating more often than usual, it could be due to elevated blood sugar levels. When your body's cells cannot absorb glucose efficiently, the kidneys try to flush it out of your system via increased urination.
- **Fatigue**: Elevated blood sugar levels can lead to fatigue because your cells are not getting enough glucose. As a result, you may experience feelings of tiredness and lack of energy.
- **Blurred vision:** High blood sugar levels can affect the tiny blood vessels in your eyes, leading to blurred or distorted vision. If you experience any changes in vision, along with other symptoms of high blood sugar, it's essential to seek medical attention.
- **Abdominal pain and vomiting**: If your blood sugar levels are severely elevated, you might experience abdominal pain, nausea, and vomiting. This situation could lead to diabetic ketoacidosis, a potentially life-threatening condition that requires immediate medical attention.

When To Go to the ER

If you experience any of the above symptoms, and they are severe and persistent, you should seek medical attention immediately.

The same advice applies if your blood sugar levels are above 240 mg/dL. At that point, it's crucial to seek medical attention. High blood sugar levels can lead to severe complications such as diabetic coma, which requires urgent medical attention. Make sure you have a plan in place in case of an emergency and know when to seek medical attention.

Signs and Symptoms of Low Blood Sugar

Managing diabetes requires a delicate balance of blood sugar levels, and when those levels drop too low, it can lead to hypoglycemia, or low blood sugar. The symptoms of low blood sugar can range from mild to severe, and it is important to recognize them and act before they become dangerous.

When your blood sugar levels are low, some of the initial signs to watch out for are sweating, trembling, and feeling dizzy. You might also feel hungry, anxious, or irritable. It is not uncommon to have a headache or to feel weak or lightheaded.

Some other signs of low blood sugar include:

- **Change in behavior**: As your blood glucose level continues to drop, you might experience sudden changes in speech or behavior, such as confusion or slurred speech. There is also a possibility of mood swings ranging from embarrassment to aggressive behavior. You might feel like a different person.
- **Physical manifestations:** If left unchecked, severe hypoglycemia can cause seizures, loss of consciousness, or even coma. At this stage, you might experience blurred or double vision. You might appear confused to others and even start making poor judgments, like being unable to tell left from right.
- **Nighttime hypoglycemia:** Low blood sugar can occur at any time of the day or night, but many people with diabetes experience nighttime hypoglycemia. Symptoms of hypoglycemia can wake you up in the middle of the night (nightmares, feeling disoriented) and interfere with your sleep and overall ability to focus. Keep a close eye on nighttime symptoms.

THE IMPORTANCE OF REGULAR MEDICAL CHECK-UPS

Medical check-ups are an essential part of diabetes management. Regular check-ups allow your doctor to monitor your blood sugar levels, blood pressure, and cholesterol.

This can help to prevent or identify complications that may arise from diabetes, such as heart disease, kidney disease, and nerve damage. Your doctor can also identify changes in your health and suggest adjustments to your diabetes management plan to keep you healthy and prevent complications.

Regular medical check-ups give you a chance to discuss any concerns or questions you may have with your doctor. This is an opportunity to review your progress, discuss your treatment plan, and make any necessary changes.

You can discuss any new symptoms you may be experiencing, and your doctor can recommend any necessary tests or referrals. This helps to ensure that you are getting the best possible care and that you are managing your diabetes effectively.

One of the benefits of regular medical check-ups is the opportunity for your doctor to screen for other health conditions that may be related to diabetes.

For example, people with type 2 diabetes are at a higher risk of developing eye conditions, such as diabetic retinopathy.

Regular eye exams can help identify any changes in your vision and prevent damage to your eyes. Your doctor can also screen for other conditions, such as infections and foot problems, which can occur more frequently in people with diabetes.

Regular medical check-ups can also help you to stay motivated and on track with your diabetes management plan.

It can be frustrating and challenging to manage diabetes, but appointments with your doctor can serve as a reminder of the progress you've made and the goals you're working towards. Your doctor can offer guidance and support and can provide you with the tools you need to stay on top of your diabetes management.

Remember that managing diabetes is a lifelong journey—regular medical check-ups are a crucial part of your diabetes management plan.

Now that we've gone over a basic exploration of your options, let's cover in more detail one of the biggest aspects of diabetes management: your diet!

5

MANAGING DIABETES THROUGH DIET

"Good food is wise medicine."

— ALISON LEVITT M.D.

You are what you eat.

There is so much truth to that statement, though of course, it can also be laughable.

You do not become a donut just because you eat a donut, and you don't become a stalk of celery because that's what you choose to snack on, either. That is obvious.

However, what many people do not realize is the major impact that diet has on our overall health. Perhaps nowhere is that truer than for the person with type 2 diabetes.

It is true that managing diabetes can be a challenge, and it's also true that some risk factors for diabetes (like your genetics) are completely out of your control.

But there are some areas in which you have total control — and can take charge of your diabetes symptoms. One of those is your diet.

As the quote above illustrates, the best medicine you can put into your body is the food you choose to nourish it with.

Managing diabetes through diet is all about making healthy choices that work for your situation. Everyone with diabetes is unique, and their dietary needs will differ.

A registered dietitian can help you develop a customized meal plan that includes the right foods in the right proportions, so I do recommend checking in with a nutritionist or dietician for a more personalized plan.

With that said, let's look at some of the most important information about diabetes and your diet so you can make the best and most informed decisions for your needs.

THE ROLE OF CARBOHYDRATES, FATS, AND PROTEINS IN BLOOD SUGAR CONTROL

Carbohydrates are often considered to be the most significant factor in blood sugar control. The carbohydrate in food breaks down into glucose, which is then absorbed into the bloodstream.

The glucose acts as fuel for the body, but in the case of people with diabetes, it can result in high levels of blood sugar.

To manage this, people with diabetes need to ensure that they are consuming the right amount of carbohydrates in their diet and avoiding foods that can spike their blood sugar levels. Ideally, people with diabetes should follow a diet that is low in simple carbohydrates, but high in complex carbohydrates such as whole grains, vegetables, and fruits.

Fats are also a key component in blood sugar control. The right balance of healthy fats can help to decrease insulin resistance and inflammation, leading to improved blood sugar levels.

However, a diet that is high in saturated and trans fats can cause inflammation and lead to insulin resistance, which can be harmful to those with diabetes. Foods that are high in healthy fats include nuts, fatty fish (such as salmon or tuna), avocados, and olive oil.

Protein is vital in maintaining muscle mass and is an excellent source of energy. However, when eating protein, people with diabetes need to exercise caution as it can raise blood sugar levels.

When consuming protein, it is essential to eat smaller portions and to balance it with fiber-rich foods such as vegetables. The best sources of protein for people with diabetes are lean meats, fish, nuts, and legumes.

RECOMMENDED DIETARY GUIDELINES

Again, one of the best ways to manage type 2 diabetes is through proper nutrition. By following recommended dietary guidelines, people with diabetes can maintain healthy blood glucose levels and reduce the risk of diabetes-related complications.

The Importance of Portion Control and Meal Planning

Portion control is key to managing blood glucose levels.

By controlling the amount of carbohydrates, protein, and fat in each meal, people with type 2 diabetes can maintain stable blood sugar levels throughout the day. Shortly, I'll introduce you to "the plate method" to help you balance your meals.

Meal planning is also an essential component of managing diabetes. Planning meals ahead of time can help people stick to their nutrition goals and avoid unhealthy food choices.

Carrying healthy snacks when on-the-go can also help prevent impulse eating and keep blood sugar levels in check.

Strategies for Eating Out and Managing Special Occasions

Eating out and attending special occasions can be challenging for people with diabetes. However, with the right strategies, it is still possible to enjoy meals and events while maintaining healthy blood glucose levels.

When eating out, it's a good idea to check the menu ahead of time and choose restaurants that offer healthy options whenever possible. Pay attention to portion sizes and limit unhealthy extras such as butter, cream, and sugar.

During special occasions such as holidays and family gatherings, it's easy to indulge in unhealthy food options. One way to avoid this is to bring a healthy dish to share. This ensures that there will be at least one healthy option available. It's also important to pace your eating and to avoid going back for seconds.

Widely Accepted Diabetes "Superfoods"

Some foods are considered "superfoods" for people with type 2 diabetes.

What is a "superfood"? It's just a food that has been shown to be particularly beneficial in managing blood glucose levels and reducing the risk of diabetes-related complications. Some of these foods include:

- Non-starchy vegetables such as broccoli, spinach, and kale

- Whole grains such as brown rice, quinoa, and barley
- Lean proteins such as chicken, fish, and tofu
- Nuts and seeds such as almonds, walnuts, and chia seeds
- Healthy fats such as olive oil, avocado, and flaxseed oil

WHAT ABOUT DIETARY SUPPLEMENTS?

As a person with type 2 diabetes, you are likely always searching for ways to manage your condition and keep your blood sugar levels in check. One potential avenue many people explore is the consumption of dietary supplements. But with so many options out there, and conflicting information about their effectiveness, it can be hard to know where to start.

First, let's define what we mean by "dietary supplements." These are products that contain one or more ingredients like vitamins, minerals, herbs, or other botanicals, amino acids, or enzymes.

They're intended to supplement the diet, and come in many forms like capsules, tablets, powders, and drinks. Some dietary supplements are marketed specifically for people with diabetes, claiming to lower blood sugar levels or improve insulin sensitivity.

For instance, magnesium has been shown in some studies to improve insulin sensitivity and glucose control, although the dosage and duration required to have an effect are still unknown.

Similarly, St. John's wort, an herb commonly used to treat depression and anxiety, has been studied for its potential to lower blood sugar levels.

Note that not all supplements are created equal, and some can even be harmful if taken in excess.

For example, high doses of vitamins like A, D, E, and K can accumulate in the body and cause toxic effects. Other supplements may interact with medications like insulin, causing adverse effects.

That is why it's essential to talk to your healthcare provider before taking any supplements, especially if you're using prescription medications or have other health conditions that could be affected.

Another thing to keep in mind is that dietary supplements are not a substitute for a healthy diet and lifestyle. As the name implies, they are meant to supplement your existing routine, not replace it. Eating a balanced diet that is rich in whole grains, fruits and vegetables, lean protein, and healthy fats, combined with regular physical activity, is still the cornerstone of diabetes management.

Finally, it's worth mentioning that dietary supplements can be costly, and insurance may not cover them. It's wise to do some research and compare prices and quality before making a purchase, and to be wary of claims that sound too good to be true.

If you do decide to try a supplement, always choose reputable brands that have been third-party tested for purity and potency and beware of products sold online or in unauthorized retail outlets.

Common supplements used in type 2 diabetes include the following:

- Vitamin B12
- Vitamin D
- Magnesium
- Zinc
- Chromium
- Alpha lipoic acid
- Coenzyme Q10

GUIDANCE ON CREATING YOUR OWN HEALTHY EATING PLAN

A carefully planned diet can help you manage your blood sugar levels, reduce the risk of complications, and improve your overall health. But with so much conflicting information out there, creating your own healthy eating plan can be overwhelming.

Here are some tips.

Why Do You Need to Develop a Healthy Eating Plan?

I'd like to begin by emphasizing why it's so important to develop a healthy eating plan in the first place.

Remember, type 2 diabetes is a chronic condition that occurs when the body becomes resistant to insulin or does not produce enough insulin. Insulin is a hormone that regulates the amount of glucose in your blood.

When your body cannot regulate blood glucose levels effectively, it can lead to a range of complications, including heart disease, stroke, nerve damage, and kidney disease. A healthy eating plan can help you manage your blood sugar levels, control your weight, and reduce your risk of complications.

What Does a Diabetes Diet Involve?

A diabetes diet involves eating a balanced and healthy diet that is low in sugar, saturated and trans fats, cholesterol, and sodium.

This means that you need to limit your intake of processed foods, sugar-sweetened beverages, and high-fat meats. Instead, your diet should consist of nutrient-dense foods, such as vegetables, fruits, whole grains, lean proteins, and healthy fats.

Recommended Foods

The following foods are recommended for people with type 2 diabetes:

- **Vegetables:** Eat a variety of non-starchy vegetables, such as broccoli, spinach, kale, carrots, and peppers.
- **Fruits**: Choose fruits that are low in sugar and high in fiber, such as berries, apples, pears, and oranges.
- **Whole grains:** Choose whole-grain bread, pasta, rice, and cereals.
- **Lean proteins**: Choose lean proteins such as skinless chicken, fish, tofu, and legumes.
- **Healthy fats:** Use olive oil, avocado, nuts, and seeds in moderation.

Foods to Avoid

The following foods should be avoided or limited:

- **Sugary drinks:** Avoid sugar-sweetened beverages such as soda, fruit juice, and sweetened tea.
- **Processed foods:** Limit your intake of processed foods such as white bread, chips, crackers, and cookies.
- **High-fat meats**: Avoid red meat, bacon, sausage, and other high-fat meats.
- **Saturated and trans fats:** Limit your intake of saturated and trans fats found in butter, cheese,

cream, and fried foods.
- **Sodium**: Limit your salt intake to less than 2,300 mg per day.

Putting it All Together: Creating a Plan

Now that you know the basics, how do you create a plan that will help you to coast through any mealtime like a champ? Here are some general ideas that can help you out as you become accustomed to eating a more wholesome, healthful diet.

The Plate Method

The plate method I mentioned earlier is a simple and effective way to plan your meals.

Start by dividing your plate into three sections: half of the plate should be filled with non-starchy vegetables, one quarter with lean protein, and one quarter with grains or starchy vegetables.

This method ensures that you have a balanced meal with carbohydrates, protein, and fiber. You can also add a small serving of fruit or dairy as a snack.

Counting Carbohydrates

Counting carbohydrates is another way to manage your blood sugar levels. Carbohydrates are essential for energy, but some types of carbohydrates can cause a spike in blood sugar levels.

It's important to choose carbohydrates that are high in fiber and avoid refined carbohydrates.

You can start by aiming for 45-60 grams of carbohydrates per meal. A registered dietitian can help you create a personalized meal plan based on your individual needs.

Choose Your Foods

When creating your healthy eating plan, focus on whole foods and avoid processed foods. Whole foods are nutrient-dense and provide your body with essential vitamins and minerals.

Processed foods, on the other hand, are often high in added sugars, sodium, and unhealthy fats. Aim for a variety of colorful vegetables, lean protein, healthy fats, and whole grains.

Glycemic Index

The glycemic index is a ranking system that measures how quickly foods raise blood sugar levels.

Foods with a high glycemic index can cause a spike in blood sugar, whole foods with a low glycemic index can help maintain a steady blood sugar level.

Choose foods with a low glycemic index, such as non-starchy vegetables, whole grains, and legumes. Avoid foods with a high glycemic index, such as processed foods, sugary drinks, and refined carbohydrates.

PUTTING TOGETHER A BASIC MENU PLAN

Need some help putting together a basic menu plan? Here's a sample of one you can use to help you guide your decisions day to day.

Remember, this isn't a "must-do" menu — it's simply some suggestions and ideas to help get you started. You can swap out these foods for ones you like, or ones you prefer to include in your diet for other reasons (for example, getting rid of the milk because you're dairy-free).

Day 1:
Breakfast: Omelet with spinach, mushrooms, and tomatoes (306 calories)
Lunch: Turkey wrap with avocado, lettuce, and tomato on a whole wheat tortilla (342 calories)
Dinner: Grilled chicken breast with steamed vegetables and brown rice (412 calories)
Snack: Greek yogurt with berries (180 calories)

Day 2:
Breakfast: Whole wheat toast with peanut butter and banana (389 calories)
Lunch: Salad with grilled shrimp, mixed greens, cherry tomatoes, and avocado (388 calories)
Dinner: Baked salmon filet with roasted asparagus and quinoa (465 calories)
Snack: Apple slices with almond butter (172 calories)

Day 3:
Breakfast: Greek yogurt with chia seeds and mixed berries (215 calories)
Lunch: Grilled chicken breast with mixed greens and cherry tomatoes (284 calories)
Dinner: Spaghetti squash with turkey bolognese sauce (345 calories)
Snack: Hard-boiled egg with carrot sticks (134 calories)

Day 4:
Breakfast: Oatmeal with sliced banana and cinnamon (268 calories)
Lunch: Tuna salad with mixed greens and avocado (321 calories)
Dinner: Pan-seared pork chops with roasted Brussels sprouts and sweet potato (471 calories)
Snack: Hummus with carrot and celery sticks (152 calories)

Day 5:
Breakfast: Scrambled eggs with cheese and spinach (346 calories)
Lunch: Grilled chicken salad with mixed greens, cherry tomatoes, and balsamic vinaigrette (244 calories)
Dinner: Grilled steak with roasted sweet potatoes and green beans (500 calories)
Snack: Blueberries with a handful of almonds (187 calories)

Day 6:
Breakfast: Veggie breakfast burrito with scrambled eggs, peppers, onions, and cheese (311 calories)
Lunch: Seafood soup with shrimp, fish, and vegetables (292 calories)
Dinner: Grilled chicken with roasted zucchini and brown rice (454 calories)
Snack: Plain Greek yogurt with sliced peaches (143 calories)

Day 7:
Breakfast: Cottage cheese with mixed berries and honey (215 calories)
Lunch: Grilled chicken with mixed greens and cherry tomatoes (284 calories)
Dinner: Baked tilapia with mixed veggies and quinoa (391 calories)
Snack: Sliced cucumber with hummus (92 calories)

All the meals mentioned above have been selected with precision and are balanced with protein, carbohydrates, and fats that will help you stay full for longer and keep your blood sugar levels in check.

Moreover, if you look closely, all the meals are nutrient-dense and include lots of fresh and wholesome ingredients, providing you with the necessary macro and micronutrients.

You may also find it helpful to use a basic calorie counting chart to keep yourself in check.

Essentially, this chart is just a table or spreadsheet where you can track the number of calories, macronutrients, and mealtimes for each of the foods you consume. You can create your chart with a pen and paper or a digital app to track it over time, for example, in your mobile phone.

Here's one I like to use:

Time	Date	Food	Calories
Total Daily Calories			

HOW TO READ AND UNDERSTAND FOOD LABELS

As you know now, knowing what to eat and what not to eat is crucial when it comes to managing your blood sugar levels. That easy when you're eating raw fruits and vegetables but what about when you are buying something off the shelves?

Understanding how to decode food labels is another important step in healthy eating to manage your type 2 diabetes. Here are some tips.

Start With the Serving Size

The serving size is displayed prominently on the top of the nutrition facts label.

Always start here because everything else on the label is based on this serving size. Most food products contain multiple servings, so it's essential to pay attention to how many servings you're consuming.

For example, if the serving size of a pack of cookies is two, but you eat the entire pack of ten, you need to increase the calories, carbs, and other nutrients listed on the label to accurately reflect your consumption.

Carb Content

When reading food labels, always check the total number of carbohydrates listed per serving size. It can be useful to compare the carb content of similar products to help you make the best choice. Look for products with fewer carbs, which can help you better manage your blood sugar levels.

Sugar and Sugar Substitutes

Many products contain added sugar, which can significantly affect your blood sugar levels. Pay attention to the total sugar content listed on the food label and avoid products with too much added sugar.

Always check the ingredient list for sugar substitutes like high fructose corn syrup, agave, or brown rice syrup. These substitutes may not spike your blood sugar as quickly as table sugar, but they can still affect your blood sugar levels.

Manufacturers sometimes use sneaky names for sugar, such as dextrose, sucrose, and maltodextrin. Watch out for other hidden ingredients too, such as trans fats, sodium, and artificial flavors and colors.

Alcohol's Effect on Glucose

Alcohol and glucose metabolism are closely linked. When you consume alcohol, your liver goes into overdrive to process it. This process slows down the release of glucose from the liver into the bloodstream, which can cause your blood sugar levels to drop. This drop can last for up to 24 hours after you've had your last drink.

As this impact on glucose control can put you at risk, it's crucial to maintain close blood glucose monitoring while drinking.

Another thing to factor in is the effect of mixers on glucose levels when drinking. If you add sugary drinks or mixers to your alcoholic drink, you're increasing your blood glucose levels with a similar effect on glucose metabolism. Mix alcohol with low or sugar-free options such as diet coke, sparkling water, or fresh citrus juices.

When planning to drink, remember that it can be a good idea to eat a meal containing complex carbohydrates like whole wheat bread, potatoes, peas, or beans. Eating these kinds of foods alongside your drink can help keep your blood sugar levels stable while you enjoy drinking.

It's advisable to monitor your blood glucose levels in the morning after a night of drinking, particularly before eating. Doing so will allow you to adjust your intake if you experience a reading that is beyond your target range.

The influence of alcohol on the glucose levels in the body can vary, so monitoring and taking slow and steady steps to adjust accordingly will be helpful in stabilizing blood sugar levels.

SMOKING AND DIABETES

Like alcohol, smoking and diabetes are two major health concerns that are also closely connected.

Smoking not only increases the risk of developing diabetes, but it can also make diabetes management more challenging. If you have type 2 diabetes, you need to take the time to understand the relationship between smoking and diabetes and take the necessary steps to quit smoking ASAP.

How Can Smoking Lead to Diabetes?

Several studies have shown that smoking results in insulin resistance, making it difficult for the body to use insulin effectively. As insulin is responsible for regulating blood sugar levels, impaired insulin function can lead to high blood sugar levels, a precursor to diabetes.

Smoking can also damage blood vessels and organs, leading to metabolic dysfunction that impairs glucose metabolism. And the list of problems doesn't end there—smoking can also increase cortisol levels, which causes high blood sugar levels.

Smoking if you have Diabetes

Smoking can make it challenging to manage diabetes and increase the complications associated with it. People with diabetes who smoke are more likely to develop cardiovascular disease, kidney disease, eye disease, and neuropathy.

Smoking narrows blood vessels, reducing blood flow to vital organs, and can cause nerve damage, which makes it difficult to feel foot injuries, infections, and wounds.

Smoking and Sleep

Smoking can also affect sleep quality, which impacts diabetes management (something I'll discuss in more detail in the next section).

People who smoke are more likely to snore and have sleep apnea. Sleep apnea can cause blood sugar levels to spike, leading to insulin resistance and making diabetes harder to manage.

Moreover, sleep-deprived individuals have impaired glucose metabolism and are more likely to make poor food choices that affect blood sugar levels.

Does Smoking Cause Diabetes?

Although smoking is not a direct cause of diabetes, it can increase the risk of developing type 2 diabetes.

Moreover, smoking can make it harder to control blood sugar levels once someone has diabetes. Smoking increases the risks of multiple health issues, and quitting smoking is an essential step toward optimal health.

Quitting Can Help

Quitting smoking is by far the most effective way to reduce the risks associated with smoking and diabetes. If you need help quitting, seek support from friends, family, or healthcare providers.

Nicotine replacement therapy, medication, and counseling can all help smokers quit smoking successfully and manage diabetes more effectively. Quitting can lower blood pressure, improve blood sugar levels, and reduce the risk of complications associated with diabetes.

SLEEP AND DIABETES

A good night's sleep doesn't just help you feel refreshed, it also helps you manage your diabetes. As someone living with diabetes, you need to understand how your sleeping habits can impact your blood sugar levels.

Sleep Can Both Raise and Lower Glucose Levels

Some individuals with diabetes may experience a rise in blood sugar levels during sleep, especially if the body releases stress hormones such as cortisol.

On the other hand, some individuals may experience a drop in blood sugar levels while sleeping, which is known as nocturnal hypoglycemia.

Therefore, it's essential to monitor your blood sugar levels regularly, especially before bedtime. You may want to consult with your doctor to adjust your medications, insulin, or diet to avoid experiencing sudden spikes or drops in your glucose levels.

Why Sleep Affects Blood Sugar

Researchers have found that lack of sleep or poor sleep quality can negatively impact insulin sensitivity, which is essential for your body to properly regulate blood sugar levels.

Moreover, a lack of sleep can increase stress hormones such as cortisol, which can lead to an increase in blood glucose levels. It's essential to aim for 7-8 hours of sleep per night to improve insulin sensitivity, avoid developing a resistant state, and lower your chances of developing type 2 diabetes complications.

Blood Sugar Levels May Also Impact Sleep Quality

On the flip side, elevated blood sugar levels can impact your sleep quality, too. Studies show that people with high blood sugar levels often experience low-quality sleep due to frequent urination, night sweats, and restless legs syndrome.

Maintaining good glycemic control is essential for achieving a restful and rejuvenating sleep. Be sure to manage your blood sugar levels during the day to enhance your chances of sleeping better at night.

Benefits of Good Quality Sleep

Getting optimal sleep every night is essential for people living with diabetes to achieve and maintain good health.

Adequate sleep has been linked to numerous benefits such as enhanced insulin sensitivity, improved blood sugar control, lowered risk of developing type 2 diabetes and its complications, reduced inflammation, lower stress levels, and enhanced mental and physical well-being.

To reap these benefits, aim for a healthy sleep schedule every night.

STRESS AND DIABETES

Stress is an inevitable part of our lives. Whether it's the stress of work, family, or finances, it takes a toll on our well-being. As a person with type 2 diabetes, you may be at a higher risk of experiencing stress-related complications. Stress can affect your blood sugar levels, making it harder to manage your diabetes.

Fortunately, there are ways to manage stress and lower your risk of developing diabetes-related complications. I won't go into too much detail here, since I'll tackle this topic in more depth later in the book.

However, for now, know that stress can affect your body in various ways. When you're stressed, your body responds by releasing stress hormones such as cortisol and adrenaline. These hormones cause your heart to beat faster, your blood pressure to rise, and your blood sugar levels to increase.

For people with diabetes, this can be particularly problematic. Chronic stress can make it harder to control your blood sugar levels, leading to long-term complications such as nerve damage and cardiovascular disease.

The first step in managing stress is to identify your triggers. What situations or events cause you the most stress? Once you've identified your triggers, come up with a plan to manage them. Some techniques that may work for you include practicing relaxation techniques such as deep breathing or meditation, exercising regularly, and talking to a trusted friend or family member.

Taking care of yourself is essential when it comes to managing stress and preventing diabetes-related complications. Make sure to get enough sleep, eat a healthy diet, and engage in activities that you enjoy. Self-care can also mean saying no to certain obligations or commitments if they're too stressful for you.

Of course, an essential part of self-care is making sure you eat a proper diet. Hopefully, you now have some good ideas of what that healthy diet might look like and ways you can start transitioning to a healthier eating plan today.

Don't beat yourself up if every meal or even every day of eating isn't perfect. There's room for enjoyment in a healthy diet if you strive toward healthy food choices 80% of the time, the remaining 20% can be left up to your own personal preference. Do your best, and you'll find that even the small changes start to add up to big results over time. Remember to keep sugar content in moderation but don't completely deprive yourself of your favorite things.

Diet is an obvious intervention for diabetes, but many people don't recognize the importance of the second most important diabetes treatment and lifestyle adjustment which is exercise.

Ready to get moving? Whether you're fond of jogging, swimming, Zumba, or powerlifting it's time to learn more about how exercise can be used to help you manage your type 2 diabetes.

EXERCISE AND PHYSICAL ACTIVITY FOR DIABETES MANAGEMENT

"I do not love to work out, but if I stick to exercising every day and put the right things in my mouth, then my diabetes just stays in check."

— HALLE BERRY

There's a saying that I like to live by on mornings where I'm finding it hard to get out of bed for my daily jog.

"A body in motion tends to stay in motion."

I've always found that after taking a few days away from my normal exercise routine, I have a really hard time getting back into it. It's very easy for a few days to turn into a few weeks, a few months, and before you know it, I'm back to being completely sedentary again.

The more I exercise, though, the easier it is for me to include it as part of my daily routine. It becomes second nature, just like brushing my teeth or taking a shower.

If you have diabetes, it's so important that exercise becomes part of your daily routine, too.

As the above quote from Haller Berry demonstrates, if you're able to prioritize your body by giving it what it needs via regular movement (and of course, the healthy diet I've already talked extensively about), you'll have a far easier time managing your diabetes than you would if you chose to live a more inactive lifestyle.

And if you're already active, diabetes shouldn't be viewed as an impediment to your active lifestyle. Just take the example of Peter Shaw, an avid kite surfer. He went out of his way to find an insulin pump with an on-board blood test meter that would allow him to continue to spend lots of time in the water (and in a wetsuit). Exercise should be part of your lifestyle, as someone with diabetes.

But why is that? And are all forms of exercise built alike in terms of their overall benefits? The answers to these questions might surprise you.

So, what are you waiting for? Lace up those sneakers and let's get a move on. It's time to learn about all the benefits associated with exercise for people with diabetes.

WHY YOU NEED TO GET ACTIVE AND START EXERCISING

When it comes to diabetes, even small amounts of exercise can make a big difference. For example, a 30-minute brisk walk after dinner can help regulate blood sugar levels and reduce the risk of complications. Exercise also helps to improve insulin sensitivity, which means your body can use insulin more efficiently.

Now that you understand the benefits of exercise, it's time to get started. If you are new to exercise, start slowly and gradually increase your activity level. Mix up your routine to keep it interesting and find activities you enjoy. Walking, swimming, dancing, and cycling are all low-impact exercises that are great for people with diabetes. Aim to be active for at least 30 minutes a day, most days of the week.

There are two types of exercise that are essential for people with diabetes: aerobic exercise and strength training.

Aerobic exercise includes things like walking, jogging, biking, or swimming which are activities you can do any day of the week. Strength training involves using weights or resistance bands to build muscle. Ideally, you should aim for two to three strength training sessions per week.

It's easy to make excuses for why you can't exercise.

For example, you may say you don't have enough time during the day or that you don't have access to a gym. But the truth is, you don't need a gym membership to be physically active.

Simple activities like taking the stairs instead of the elevator, walking your dog, or doing some light stretching while watching TV can all help to increase your daily activity. It's also important to schedule your exercise into your day and make it a priority. Treat your exercise time like an appointment that can't be missed.

When it comes to staying motivated, turning your excuses into solutions is key. If you have trouble finding a long block of time for exercise, try breaking it up into smaller increments throughout the day.

Maybe you can take a 10-minute walk during your lunch break or walk around your house during commercial breaks while watching TV.

Another plan is to buddy up with a friend or family member who also wants to be active. Having someone to exercise with can be more enjoyable and hold you accountable.

Remember to track your progress and celebrate your successes, no matter how small. This can help keep you motivated and remind you why you started in the first place.

DIABETES AND EXERCISE: WHEN TO MONITOR YOUR BLOOD SUGAR

It's important to keep in mind that your blood sugar levels can be impacted by movement, especially at first, if your body isn't quite used to it yet.

Below, I'll give you some general guidelines on how and when to check your blood sugar levels as part of your fitness routine.

Recommended Exercise Guidelines

It's essential to monitor your blood sugar levels before exercising, especially if you take insulin or other diabetes medications. This can help you determine whether you need to adjust your medication dosage or eat a snack to avoid hypoglycemia (low blood sugar).

If your blood sugar is too high, it's best to wait until it's back to a healthy range before beginning exercise.

You should also check your blood sugar levels every 30 minutes during exercise, especially if you're new to exercise, trying a new activity, or exercising for an extended period. This can help you determine whether you need to reduce the intensity of your workout, take a break, or eat a snack to avoid hypoglycemia.

If your blood sugar is too low, stop exercising, and eat a small snack or drink some juice to bring your levels back up.

And after exercise, checking your blood sugar levels can help you determine how your body responds to exercise and whether you need to make any adjustments to your diabetes management plan. If your blood sugar levels are too low, eat a snack or drink some juice to bring them back up. If your blood sugar levels are too high, it's essential to monitor them closely and possibly adjust your diabetes medication dosage or diet plan.

DIFFERENT TYPES OF EXERCISE AND HOW THEY AFFECT BLOOD SUGAR

Aerobic exercises such as brisk walking, cycling, and swimming can help your body use insulin efficiently and lower your blood sugar levels. During aerobic exercise, your heart rate increases, and your muscles use more glucose for energy.

This increases the number of insulin receptors your cells need to uptake insulin. This type of exercise is good for those with diabetes because it can help reduce the amount of medications or even insulin injections needed. Aim for 150 minutes of moderate-intensity aerobic activity per week and break this down into at least 30 minutes, 5 days a week.

Strength training exercises such as lifting weights, resistance band exercises and Pilates are also good for those with type 2 diabetes. Strength training can be an effective way to improve insulin sensitivity and decrease blood sugar levels.

If you can, you should perform these exercises at least two days a week, allowing 48 hours between workouts.

Aerobics and strength-training are the two most common "categories" of exercise, but there are a few other varieties to keep in mind as well.

One is HIIT. High-Intensity Interval Training is a type of exercise that involves short periods of intense activity followed by a short period of rest or a slower activity. This type of exercise has been shown to improve blood sugar control and lower A1C levels in those with type 2 diabetes. It can be challenging, so it's essential to listen to your body and consult with a healthcare professional before starting.

Flexibility training or stretching exercises such as yoga are good for maintaining mobility, stability, and balance. These exercises can improve blood glucose levels indirectly by reducing stress levels and boosting your metabolism. You can stretch for a few minutes every day or incorporate yoga classes into your exercise routine.

Finally, mind-body exercises such as tai chi and qigong are great for reducing stress levels and improving blood sugar levels. These types of exercises focus on meditation, deep breathing, and slow, flowing movements that can help decrease blood pressure and improve feelings of well-being.

SAFETY CONSIDERATIONS FOR EXERCISE WITH DIABETES

Exercise plays an essential role in the management of diabetes. However, exercise-induced hypoglycemia is one of the significant concerns people with diabetes face. Exercise can make it challenging to maintain blood glucose levels during and after physical activity.

In addition to regularly checking and monitoring your blood sugar levels, as mentioned earlier, there are some basic safety tips you'll want to follow.

For starters, you should always carry a source of glucose with you, such as candies, glucose tablets, or a sports drink. If you experience symptoms of hypoglycemia, you can consume these drinks to bring your blood glucose levels back to normal.

If you are new to exercising, it's recommended to start with low-intensity exercises and gradually increase the intensity levels. Sudden and drastic changes to your exercise routine can affect your blood glucose levels and can be a potential risk for hypoglycemia. Always consult with your doctor before starting any exercise routine.

Always keep a record of your workout routine, blood glucose levels, and any other relevant information. This helps you identify how different exercises affect your glucose levels. You can make the necessary adjustments to your diet, medication, and exercise routine to maintain healthy glucose levels.

Keeping yourself hydrated is also smart, especially when you are exercising. Dehydration can affect your glucose levels and lead to potential risks. Drink plenty of fluids before, during, and after exercise. Remember to always keep a water bottle with you during workouts.

IMPORTANCE OF INCORPORATING PHYSICAL ACTIVITY INTO YOUR DAILY LIFE

At this point, I hope you're convinced that the benefits of regular physical activity are numerous, particularly for people with type 2 diabetes. In addition to improving insulin sensitivity and glycemic control, suitable physical activity can reduce blood pressure, improve cholesterol levels, and increase cardiovascular health.

Moreover, regular exercise can benefit your mental health by reducing anxiety and depression levels, boosting mood, and improving sleep quality.

However, even with all the benefits that come with exercise, it can be difficult to get started or stay motivated.

Be patient with yourself and remember to consult your doctor before starting a new routine. By setting achievable goals and taking things one day at a time, you'll not only help to alleviate some of the symptoms of your type 2 diabetes, but you may be able to prevent further complications from taking hold.

Having covered these basic lifestyle adjustments as the first line treatments for managing diabetes, let's move on to ways you can prevent possible (and potentially major) complications that might come about because of diabetes.

7

MANAGING TYPE 2 DIABETES COMPLICATIONS

"Trying to manage diabetes is hard because if you don't, there are consequences you'll have to deal with later in life."

— BRYAN ADAMS

Living with type 2 diabetes can feel like a full-time job. It can be tough to deal with the balancing act of managing blood sugar levels while also preventing complications, but this is something that you've got to prioritize if you want to stay healthy and well.

It's not always the most fun. And it can be overwhelming!

But living with type 2 diabetes isn't just about avoiding and managing systems of the diabetes itself, but also preventing future complications. This chapter won't be the sunniest or the most cheerful, but it's important to understand potential outcomes of this disease if you want to avoid them.

Let's take a closer look at some of the most common complications of type 2 diabetes and how they can be avoided.

WHAT ARE THE RISKS OF UNCONTROLLED GLUCOSE COMPLICATIONS?

If you have type 2 diabetes, you already know that managing your blood sugar levels is imperative.

But did you know that uncontrolled blood sugar levels can lead to several serious complications? Don't panic just yet. With the right treatment and prevention strategies, you can keep these common complications at bay.

Awareness and education are key to helping you manage your diabetes and prevent future issues. If you take home anything from this book, let this be it!

I want to give you an overview of some common complications, not to scare you, but to keep you informed of potential risks so that you can take steps to actively avoid them.

Increased Risk of Heart Disease

One of the most significant problems associated with elevated blood glucose levels is an increased risk of heart disease. This is because high levels of glucose in the blood can damage the blood vessels and arteries, making it easier for plaque to build up and leading to the narrowing of the arteries.

Over time, this can reduce blood flow to your heart, leading to chest pain, heart attack, or stroke. It's essential to keep your blood glucose levels under control to reduce your risk of heart disease and other related problems.

Kidney Problems

When your blood sugar levels are uncontrolled, your kidneys must work overtime to filter out waste from your body. When your blood glucose levels are consistently high, it can lead to damage to the tiny blood vessels in your kidneys. This can lead to kidney damage or even kidney failure if left untreated.

To avoid this, make sure to control your blood sugar levels through a healthy diet, exercise, and medication as prescribed by your doctor. It's also important to keep an eye on your blood pressure and cholesterol levels, as high levels of these can also damage your kidneys.

Diabetes is the leading cause of kidney failure, so it's crucial to keep a close eye on your blood glucose levels to protect your kidneys and overall health. If you're experiencing symptoms such as increased urination, fatigue, or swelling in your legs and ankles, consult your doctor immediately.

Eye Problems

High blood glucose levels can also impact the small blood vessels in your eyes, leading to a variety of eye problems. These problems can include everything from minor changes in vision, to more complex issues such as glaucoma, cataracts, and diabetic retinopathy, and even permanent vision loss.

By keeping your blood glucose levels under control, and within a healthy range, you can help manage the progression of these issues and potentially even prevent them altogether.

It's also important to get regular eye exams from an optometrist or ophthalmologist. If you're experiencing symptoms such as eye pain, redness, or sudden changes in vision, seek medical attention right away.

Just look at the example of Rachael, a chiropractic office assistant and virtual assistant for the diabetes health coaching service Needles and Spoons.

Rachael has type 1 diabetes, so the story here is a bit different than the journey someone might experience with type 2 diabetes. Nevertheless, the potential risks and outcomes are the same.

Rachael was diagnosed with diabetes at the age of just four years old. She had managed the disease all her childhood and most of her adult life, until one day, when she was watching television with her husband, she noticed a spot in her vision. After having it checked out, she discovered she had bleeding in her retina. At the age of just 29 years old, she was legally blind.

The takeaway here is that it is so important to keep up with your eye appointments. Make sure your optometrist checks your vision and takes detailed photographs of your retinas. If you aren't happy with your eye care, get a new doctor. Diabetic retinopathy can happen to anyone, but with the right prevention and medical care, you can avoid or manage it should it happen to you.

Metabolic Syndrome

Metabolic syndrome is a group of conditions that increase your risk of heart disease, stroke, and diabetes. These conditions include increased waistline, high blood pressure, increased blood sugar, and obesity. Uncontrolled glucose levels exacerbate this risk by damaging your blood vessels and reducing insulin sensitivity. Symptoms include fatigue, pain, depressed mood, anxiety, and stress. Prevention and treatment strategies include controlling your glucose levels, managing your weight, and engaging in regular exercise.

Dementia

Studies have shown that people with type 2 diabetes are at a higher risk of developing dementia as they age. Dementia is a term given to a group of symptoms related to cognitive decline, such as memory loss and difficulty in communicating.

While the exact reasons for the link between diabetes and dementia are still unclear, researchers suggest that high glucose levels damage blood vessels in the brain, leading to cognitive problems such as memory loss, reduced ability to organize, confusion, disorientation, and changes in personality.

To minimize the risk of dementia, it's important to keep your glucose levels under control, exercise regularly, and maintain a healthy diet.

Sexual Dysfunction

Sexual health is also impacted by uncontrolled glucose levels. High glucose levels can lead to nerve and blood vessel damage, which can result in erectile dysfunction in men, and decreased sexual response and lubrication in women.

These sexual problems can seriously affect your quality of life and your relationship. Talking to your healthcare provider about these issues can help you get the appropriate treatment.

Neuropathic Pain

People with diabetes often experience neuropathic pain, which is a result of nerve damage. This commonly affects the feet and legs, but it can impact other areas of the body as well.

Uncontrolled glucose levels can worsen this pain, making it difficult to move around and perform daily activities.

Symptoms of neuropathy often include numbness, tingling, and even a sense of burning or pain. Neuropathy can also impact your ability to feel changes in temperature or pressure, which can lead to more serious problems, such as foot ulcers and infections.

Neuropathic pain can be a challenge to treat, but there are several interventions including various medications and complementary therapies that can alleviate the symptoms. Therapies and interventions include physical therapy, diabetic shoes or orthotics, TENS unit use, and acupuncture. Typical anti-inflammatory drugs and pain relief do not treat nerve pain and it is irreversible damage. The best way to treat neuropathic pain is to prevent it from happening. Anti-seizure drugs and some anti-depressants are used to help with neuropathic pain. Topical pain medications and supplements such as B vitamins, alpha lipoic acid, and acetyl-L-carnitine are often used to help with neuropathy.

Poor Wound Healing

One of the immediate and most obvious risks of uncontrolled glucose levels is poor wound healing. This presents as wounds that are difficult to close, where the skin has trouble reconnecting and closing over the wound. People with Type 2 diabetes are at an increased risk of developing cuts, bruises, and other injuries.

When blood glucose levels aren't adequately managed, the immune system is weakened, inhibiting the body's natural ability to heal. This can lead to more serious infections, a longer recovery time, and, in some cases, amputation.

Diabetic patients should see a podiatrist and have their feet checked regularly for poor healing ulcers and wounds. Wounds can occur anywhere but in patients with neuropathy they lose feeling in their feet and don't realize they have developed sores.

Immune Function Issues

As mentioned earlier, uncontrolled glucose levels also impact your immune function. When the body can't process glucose correctly, it can't produce enough energy for the cells, leading to decreased levels of white blood cells. This means that your body is more susceptible to infections and diseases.

Poor Circulation

High blood sugars can lead to a plaque buildup in your arteries. This restricts blood flow to various organs, which can cause systemic issues such as neuropathy, kidney disease, and heart disease. Poor circulation also affects the duration taken for a wound to heal, leading to more complications.

Trouble Breathing

While it's not widely known, Type 2 diabetes can increase the risk of lung diseases like asthma and chronic obstructive pulmonary disease (COPD). High blood sugar levels have been linked to reduced lung function, making breathing difficult, especially during and after exercise.

It's also possible that uncontrolled glucose levels can cause inflammation in the lungs, which can lead to these issues.

Increased Risk of Heart Disease

One of the most significant problems associated with elevated blood glucose levels is an increased risk of heart disease. This is because high levels of glucose in the blood can damage the blood vessels and arteries, making it easier for plaque to build up and leading to the narrowing of the arteries.

Over time, this can reduce blood flow to your heart, leading to chest pain, heart attack, or stroke. It's essential to keep your blood glucose levels under control to reduce your risk of heart disease and other related problems.

Cancer

People with Type 2 diabetes are at an increased risk of several types of cancer, including liver, pancreatic, and colon cancer. Although researchers aren't yet sure why this is the case, it's believed that elevated glucose levels might be a contributory factor.

As you can see, high blood glucose levels are no joke. They can lead to a variety of serious health problems that can significantly impact your quality of life. That's why it's so important to stay on top of your blood glucose levels and work with your healthcare team to manage your diabetes effectively.

Knowledge is Power

This last chapter may seem a bit bleak, and while it's not my goal to scare you or send you into a panic, I do think it's important to highlight some of the risks of type 2 diabetes. It's a serious condition, and as such, it's one you need to *take* seriously.

The good news is that there are plenty of steps you can take to manage your type 2 diabetes, some of which we've already covered in this book and involve basic lifestyle modifications.

And when those aren't enough, there's medication. Mainstream medicine is a beautiful thing and has brought us many ways to both treat and manage type 2 diabetes. Let us take a closer look at what some of these options are.

8

THE ROLE OF MEDICATIONS IN TYPE 2 DIABETES MANAGEMENT

"Laughter is the best medicine—unless you're diabetic, then insulin comes pretty high on the list."

— JASPER CARROTT

I promised a more lighthearted chapter, and here it is.

We all know that diabetes is no laughing matter. However, as something you must live with, it's important to have a good sense of humor, hence, the quote I included above. Make sure you have your medications under control before you start your standup comedy tour, please.

There are a few different types and classes of medications that can be used to treat type 2 diabetes and its symptoms. Obviously, lifestyle modifications are a huge part of managing disease, but medications also play an integral role.

In this chapter, I'd like to break those medications down a bit for you. Whether you've already been prescribed with one of them and are curious about how exactly it works or if you haven't yet talked to your doctor about which medications might be right for you it's my hope that this chapter can help clear things up for you.

Let's look, shall we?

TYPES OF MEDICATIONS FOR BLOOD SUGAR CONTROL

Managing blood sugar levels is crucial for people with type 2 diabetes. The good news is that there are different types of medications available to help in controlling blood sugar levels. However, the wide variety of options can leave you wondering which medication suits you best.

Some of the following information may be a review of what we covered earlier in this book, but I'm including it here again to make sure everything is crystal clear for you. If you have any questions, be sure to talk to your doctor for more information.

One more note before I dive into the nitty gritty of which options are available, all drugs do have the risk for side effects. Though most of these side effects are minor and are not life-threatening, it's important to be aware of them. I've detailed them below.

If you experience side effects with any of these drugs that are interfering with your quality of life, be sure to ask your doctor if there are alternative drugs that might be used in their place.

Insulin

If you've read through the earlier chapters, you'll already know that insulin is a hormone produced by the pancreas to regulate blood sugar levels. However, people with type 2 diabetes do not produce enough insulin, or their bodies have become resistant to insulin, requiring injections to regulate their blood sugar levels. There are various forms of insulin that cater to different needs.

Short-Acting Insulin

Short-acting insulin (also called regular insulin) is taken before meals to help control blood sugar spikes. This insulin works in about 30 minutes after injections, peaks in 2-3 hours, and lasts 3-6 hours. Examples include Human Regular (Humulin R, Novolin R).

Rapid-Acting Insulin

Rapid-acting insulin is taken before meals and begins working much faster than short-acting insulin. This insulin works about 15 minutes after injection and peaks in 1-2 hours, providing insulin coverage for 2-4 hours. Examples include insulin aspart (Fiasp, Novolog), insulin glulisine (Apidra) and insulin lispro (Admelog, Humalog, Lyumjev).

Intermediate-Acting Insulin

Intermediate-acting insulin takes longer to start working and lasts longer than rapid-acting insulin, making it a good option for overnight periods. This insulin takes effect 2-4 hours after injection, peaks in 4-12 hours, and is effective for 12-18 hours. Examples include NPH insulins (Humulin N, Novolin N, ReliOn).

Long-Acting Insulin

Long-acting insulin lasts for a full 24 hours and should be taken once a day. This insulin takes several hours to take effect and provides glucose lowering for 24 hours. Examples include Insulin degludec (Tresiba), detemir (Levemir), and glargine (Basaglar and Lantus).

Ultra Long-Acting Insulin

Ultra long-acting insulin reaches the blood stream in 6 hours, does not peak, and lasts 36 hours or longer. One example is insulin glargine U-300 (Toujeo).

Premixed (Combination) Insulins

Not everyone with diabetes requires insulin injections, however. For those who have lower daily insulin requirements, there are other options available, such as premixed (combination) insulins.

As the name suggests, these are a mixture of two different types of insulin that provide both a rapid and long-acting treatment in a single injection. This includes insulin 70/30, although you won't see these as often anymore.

Amylinomimetic Injectables

Amylinomimetic injectables, also referred to as amylinomimetic hormones, work differently than insulin. They work to suppress glucagon, a hormone that raises blood sugar levels, and thus lower blood sugar overall.

They are usually taken in combination with insulin injections and work to decrease the amount of insulin needed overall. One example is Symlin.

SGLT2 Inhibitor Drugs

These drugs are fairly new and are a class of medication used to help lower blood sugar levels in people with type 2 diabetes. How do they work?

SGLT2 inhibitors function by blocking the SGLT2 protein in the kidneys. This protein is responsible for reabsorbing glucose into the bloodstream from the kidneys. By blocking this protein, glucose is instead excreted through urine, leading to lower blood sugar levels.

Canagliflozin

Canagliflozin is sold under the brand name Invokana. Canagliflozin has been shown to lower A1C levels (a blood test that measures average blood sugar levels over a 3-month period) by 0.8-1.0%. Potential side effects include genital yeast infections and urinary tract infections.

Dapagliflozin

Dapagliflozin, or Farxiga, has been found to lower A1C levels by 0.6-0.7% and has the added bonus of potentially aiding in weight loss. However, like canagliflozin, urinary tract and genital infections are potential side effects.

Empagliflozin

Empagliflozin, or Jardiance, is another type of SGLT2 inhibitor. Compared to canagliflozin and dapagliflozin, empagliflozin has been found to have a greater impact on reducing the risk of heart disease in people with type 2 diabetes. Empagliflozin has also been shown to lower A1C levels by 0.6-0.7%.

Ertugliflozin

Finally, there's ertugliflozin, which is sold under the brand name Steglatro. Ertugliflozin has been found to lower A1C levels by 0.7-0.9% and can be taken alone or in combination with other diabetes medications. Like the other SGLT2 inhibitors, potential side effects include urinary tract and genital infections.

Biguanides

This drug works mainly by reducing the amount of glucose produced by your liver and helps improve insulin sensitivity. Metformin is the most commonly prescribed biguanide. It has a low risk of hypoglycemia, which makes it safe for use. It also helps with weight loss, making it an ideal option for people who need to lose weight while managing their diabetes.

Alpha-Glucosidase Inhibitors

Next up, we have alpha-glucosidase inhibitors. These drugs slow down the digestion of carbohydrates in the intestine, which reduces the amount of glucose released into the bloodstream after a meal.

Acarbose and miglitol are the two most used alpha-glucosidase inhibitors. These drugs, however, come with some gastrointestinal side effects, including bloating, diarrhea, and gas.

Dopamine-2 Agonists

Moving ahead, let's explore dopamine-2 agonists. These drugs work by increasing insulin sensitivity by affecting dopamine receptors found in the brain.

By doing so, they help reduce glucose production and help increase insulin sensitivity. Bromocriptine is the commonly used dopamine-2 agonist. It helps reduce fasting blood sugar levels without causing hypoglycemia or weight gain. An example is Cycloset (bromocriptine).

Dipeptidyl Peptidase-4 Inhibitors

These drugs work by blocking the action of the DPP-4 enzyme, which enhances insulin secretion. Sitagliptin and linagliptin are commonly used DPP-4 inhibitors. These drugs come with few side effects but must be used with caution in people with kidney disease. Examples include Januvia (sitagliptin), Onglyza (saxagliptin), Tradjenta (linagliptin), and Nesina (alogliptin).

Glucagon-Like Peptide-1 Receptor Agonists

This class of medication works by mimicking the body's natural hormone, GLP-1, which helps stimulate insulin secretion and lower glucose levels. GLP-1 agonists are available in both injectable and oral forms.

While they are effective in managing blood sugar levels, they can also come with some side effects such as nausea, vomiting, and diarrhea. Some examples of GLP-1 agonists include Byetta (twice daily) or weekly Bydureon (exenatide), Victoza (liraglutide), Trulicity (dulaglutide), Ozempic (semaglutide), and Rybelsus (oral semaglutide).

Meglitinides

Meglitinides are a type of medication that stimulates insulin release from the pancreas. They are taken orally before meals and work quickly to lower blood sugar levels. These medications can be effective for people who struggle with post-meal blood sugar spikes.

Examples of meglitinides include Prandin (repaglinide) and Starlix (nateglinide).

Sulfonylureas

Sulfonylureas have been around for over half a century and are still commonly used as a treatment for type 2 diabetes. They work by stimulating insulin secretion from the pancreas. Sulfonylureas are taken orally and are known to be very effective in lowering blood sugar levels.

However, they can also lead to weight gain and hypoglycemia. Common sulfonylureas include glipizide (Glucotrol), glimepiride (Amaryl), and glyburide (Diabeta).

Thiazolidinediones

TZDs are a type of medication that works by improving the body's sensitivity to insulin, which helps to control blood sugar levels. They are taken orally once a day and are effective in improving insulin resistance.

However, TZDs can also have some side effects such as fluid retention and an increased risk of fractures. Examples of

TZDs include pioglitazone (Actos) and rosiglitazone (Avandia).

WHICH OTHER MEDICATIONS CAN INTERFERE WITH DIABETES MEDICATIONS?

If you have type 2 diabetes and are taking medication to manage it, it's important to know that there are a few different medications that can interfere with your prescribed treatment.

And did you know that even certain over-the-counter medications can interfere with your diabetes medication? Yes, you read that right! These medications can affect your blood sugar levels and hinder your ability to control your diabetes.

Always talk to your doctor before taking *anything*, but here are some common medications that are known to interfere with diabetes treatments (I've included both OTC and prescription medications, for reference).

Pain Killers

Painkillers such as ibuprofen (Advil, Motrin) and codeine can raise blood glucose levels by blocking the effect of insulin. These medications are commonly used to manage pain and inflammation associated with arthritis, headaches, and menstrual cramps. It's essential to read the label carefully before taking these medications and consult your doctor if you're unsure about the potential risks.

Decongestants

Decongestants such as pseudoephedrine (Sudafed) and phenylephrine (found in many cough and cold products) are commonly used to treat cold and allergy symptoms. These medications can raise blood glucose levels by stimulating the liver to produce more glucose. It is recommended to avoid these medications altogether or take them under medical supervision.

Cough Syrups

Cough syrups containing sugar can significantly raise blood glucose levels. Moreover, coughing spells increase the body's demand for glucose, making it harder to manage blood sugar levels. It is advisable to opt for sugar-free cough syrups or those sweetened with alternative sweeteners. Look for cough syrups marked sugar free.

Anti-Diarrheal Medication

Anti-diarrheal medication such as loperamide (Imodium) can slow down the digestion process, leading to high blood sugar levels. Additionally, diarrhea can cause dehydration, making it harder to manage your blood sugar levels. If you need to take anti-diarrheal medication, make sure to monitor your blood sugar levels closely and drink plenty of fluids to stay hydrated.

Weight Loss Medication

Some weight loss medications, such as orlistat (Alli), can interfere with the body's ability to absorb fat-soluble vitamins and reduce insulin sensitivity. These effects can contribute to increased blood glucose levels and delay the management of diabetes.

Consult your doctor before taking any weight loss medication and shorten the duration of treatment to avoid adverse effects.

Steroids

Whether you're taking steroids (prednisone) for allergies, inflammation, or some other condition, they can interfere with diabetes medications by raising your blood sugar levels. So, if you're taking steroids, you may need to adjust your diabetes medications by talking to your doctor.

Beta Blockers

Beta blockers (metoprolol, propranolol, atenolol, carvedilol) are commonly used for high blood pressure and heart disease. However, they can also mask the symptoms of low blood sugar, which is a problem for people with diabetes who need to be able to recognize low blood sugar. If you're on beta blockers, talk to your doctor about how to monitor your blood sugar.

Diuretics

Diuretics (furosemide, torsemide, bumetanide) are used to treat conditions like high blood pressure and heart failure. However, they can also affect your blood sugar levels by increasing the amount of glucose your kidneys excrete. This can lead to high blood sugar levels. Again, talk to your doctor about adjusting your diabetes medication if you're taking diuretics.

Antipsychotics

Antipsychotic medications (risperidone, lurasidone, aripiprazole) are sometimes used to treat mental health conditions like schizophrenia and bipolar disorder. However, they can also cause weight gain, which can make it more difficult to manage diabetes. If you're taking antipsychotic medication, talk to your doctor about a plan to manage your weight.

Certain Antibiotics

Some antibiotics, like ciprofloxacin and levofloxacin, can lower blood sugar levels. This might be a good thing if you have high blood sugar, but if you're on other diabetes medications, it can be a problem. Always tell your doctor and pharmacist if you're taking these antibiotics and ask them if you need to adjust your diabetes medication.

BENEFITS AND RISKS OF MEDICATION THERAPY

First things first: Let's talk a little bit about the benefits and risks of medication therapy for type 2 diabetes. On the one hand, medications like metformin and insulin can help regulate blood sugar levels, reduce your risk of heart attack and stroke, and even improve symptoms of depression.

On the other hand, they can also cause side effects like nausea, dizziness, and gastrointestinal problems. If you're experiencing side effects from your medication, talk to your doctor. They may be able to adjust your dose or switch you to a different type of medication.

Another important thing to keep in mind is that different types of diabetes medications have different activation mechanisms.

For example, metformin works by reducing the amount of glucose produced by the liver and improving the body's sensitivity to insulin. Sulfonylureas, on the other hand, work by stimulating insulin production in the pancreas.

Depending on your individual needs and health history, your doctor may recommend one type of medication over another. If your medication isn't working as well as you'd like, it may be worth discussing alternative treatment options with your doctor.

WHAT TO DO IF YOUR DIABETES MEDICATION ISN'T WORKING

If you're concerned that your diabetes medication isn't working as well as it should be, don't hesitate to talk to your doctor. Your healthcare provider can run blood tests to assess your blood sugar levels and evaluate the effectiveness of your medication.

Depending on the results, they may recommend adjusting your dose, switching to a different medication, or offering additional support and resources to help you better manage your diabetes.

LIFESTYLE CHANGES VS MEDICATION: WHICH IS BEST?

Neither. Honestly, managing diabetes well involves an integrated approach that includes both lifestyle changes *and* medication.

Managing your diabetes isn't just about taking medication—it's also about making lifestyle changes that support your health and well-being.

Eating a nutritious diet, getting regular exercise, and managing stress can all play a role in keeping your blood sugar levels in check.

If you're struggling to adopt healthy behaviors, consider working with a registered dietitian, a personal trainer, or a mental health professional who can provide guidance and support.

THE COST OF INSULIN

If you ask somebody living with type 2 diabetes what the biggest challenges of managing their condition are, more than likely, the sky-high price of insulin will be at the top of that list. If you're one of those people, you've probably found yourself grappling with questions like: Why does insulin have to be so expensive? How can I afford to keep paying for it? And what happens if I can't?

The average price of insulin continues to rise, and while many drug manufacturers have capped their costs for consumers, it's still pricey—often more than $100 per month (with insurance).

The first thing you should do if you're struggling to keep up with the cost of insulin is talk to your doctor. While they might not be able to lower the price, they might be able to help you find affordable alternatives.

For example, there are insulin brands that are less expensive than others, and they may know which ones are covered by your insurance. There are also programs that offer financial assistance for people who can't afford insulin, and your doctor can help connect you with them.

You might also be surprised to learn that the cost of insulin can vary from one pharmacy to another. That's why it's a good idea to shop around and compare prices before filling your prescription if you are paying cash or using a discount card. Some pharmacies have their own discount cards developed to really help control costs.

Depending on your health insurance coverage, you might be able to switch to a high-deductible plan that has lower monthly premiums. Although you'll pay more out of pocket when you refill your insulin, you might end up saving money overall. Just be sure to talk with your doctor first to make sure that switching plans doesn't negatively affect your treatment.

WHY IT'S SO IMPORTANT TO STICK TO YOUR MEDICATION SCHEDULE

Managing diabetes is no walk in the park. It's a full-time job and takes a ton of discipline and focus. Having type 2 diabetes involves a lot of work, including regular visits to the endocrinologist, making lifestyle changes to better control your blood sugar levels, and of course, taking your prescribed medication on time, every time.

That might seem like tough work, but it is necessary to keep symptoms at bay and avoid further health complications. Your prescription drugs step in and control the amount of glucose in your bloodstream to maintain healthy levels.

Skipping doses can worsen or enhance your symptoms, depending on the situation, and it can throw your system off.

When your blood sugar levels are out of control, complications such as kidney disease, nerve damage, and vision problems can appear. Sticking to the prescribed medication is essential to prevent these severe complications from occurring.

As you know by now, from reading this book, the science of diabetes isn't cookie-cutter. The treatments and lifestyle changes that work for one person might not work as well for the next. While talking to your doctor about different medication options is always smart, it's also important to recognize that there are some strong mental and emotional factors that come into play when managing your type 2 diabetes.

If you don't recognize the ways in which diabetes affects your mental health, as well as your physical health, you can't be successful in managing it. In the next chapter, we'll take a closer look at some of the mental and emotional factors related to diabetes —and what you can do to manage those experiences, too.

9

MENTAL HEALTH AND EMOTIONAL WELL-BEING WITH DIABETES

"You can take hold of the situation. I feel great now. I live the right way. I wear fierce clothes. Everything I do now, I do it proud. I am a diabetic!"

— PATTI LABELLE

Living with type 2 diabetes can be challenging, but it doesn't have to be a dark cloud. Just like any other chronic illness, it presents a lifestyle change that requires focus and dedication. But it's important to remember that diabetes is not just about blood sugar levels and medication.

Managing your mental health and emotional well-being plays a vital role in your overall health and can help with managing your diabetes.

As Patti LaBelle said in her quote, you can take hold of the situation and live fiercely, even with diabetes. And part of that involves managing your mental health and emotional well-being.

In this next chapter, I'll give you some tips to help you navigate the emotional ups and downs of living with diabetes.

EMOTIONAL IMPACT OF A DIABETES DIAGNOSIS

I've noted several times that living with diabetes can be overwhelming. Suddenly, your life is filled with counting carbs, monitoring blood glucose levels, and worrying about potential complications.

All these responsibilities, on top of the emotional burden of a chronic illness, can be a lot to handle. It's important to acknowledge the emotional impact of a diabetes diagnosis and take steps to reduce stress and maintain your mental health.

How is Diabetes Linked to Emotion?

Managing diabetes can be frustrating, and it can make you feel as though your life is out of your hands. This lack of control can lead to feelings of anxiety and depression.

And what many people don't realize is that diabetes can affect your mood directly. It's not uncommon to experience mood swings because of fluctuating blood glucose levels. High blood sugar can cause irritability and fatigue, while low blood sugar can cause confusion, dizziness, and even seizures.

How Can I Reduce Stress in My Life?

Stress can cause blood sugar levels to rise, which can make managing diabetes more difficult. It's important to find healthy ways to cope with stress, such as exercise, meditation, or talking with a friend. It can also be helpful to limit your exposure to stressors in your life, such as negative news or toxic relationships.

Remember, self-care isn't selfish it's essential for maintaining your physical and emotional health.

Another way to reduce stress is to simplify your diabetes management routine. Talk to your healthcare provider about tools and resources that can make your life easier, such as a continuous glucose monitor or an insulin pump.

These devices can help take some of the burden off you and allow you to focus on living your life.

What Are the Symptoms of Depression?

It's not uncommon to experience feelings of sadness or anxiety after a diabetes diagnosis. However, if these feelings persist for more than a few weeks or begin to interfere with your daily life, you may be experiencing depression. Symptoms of depression can include:

- Persistent sadness or irritability
- Loss of interest in activities you once enjoyed
- Changes in appetite or weight
- Fatigue or loss of energy
- Difficulty sleeping or oversleeping
- Feelings of worthlessness or guilt

If you're experiencing any of these symptoms, it's important to speak with your healthcare provider. They can refer you to a mental health professional or provide other forms of support.

STRATEGIES FOR COPING WITH THE EMOTIONAL AND PSYCHOLOGICAL CHALLENGES OF DIABETES

Stress is a major contributor to high blood sugar levels, and diabetes management in and of itself can be very stressful, too.

Mindfulness and meditation can help you manage your stress levels and improve your mental wellbeing. Taking just a few minutes a day to focus on your breath and shift your attention away from your worries can have a huge impact on your diabetes management.

You may also want to consider setting some realistic goals. It's easy to get overwhelmed when you're trying to manage your diabetes. Setting unrealistic goals can make things even harder. Instead, focus on setting achievable goals and taking small steps towards them.

Celebrate your successes, no matter how small they may seem. Remember, any progress is progress.

Practicing gratitude can also help you shift your focus from what is going wrong to what is going right. It is easy to get bogged down by the challenges of living with diabetes, but taking time to recognize what you are grateful for can help you stay positive.

Start a gratitude journal, where you write down the things you are thankful for each day. Or take a few minutes each morning to reflect on what you are grateful for.

Finally, if you are finding it difficult to cope with the emotional and psychological challenges of type 2 diabetes, don't be afraid to seek professional help. Seeing a therapist or counselor can be incredibly helpful in managing stress and dealing with depression and anxiety. A healthcare professional can also help you to manage the physical aspects of your diabetes management.

IMPORTANCE OF SEEKING SUPPORT

Living with diabetes can feel isolating, but having a dedicated support system can help you stay motivated and positive. Talk to your friends and family about your challenges and let them help you.

Joining a diabetes support group or finding an online community can also be incredibly helpful. Surrounding yourself with people who understand what you are going through can make all the difference in the world.

Understanding Fact vs. Myth

There is a lot of misinformation out there about type 2 diabetes, which can make it difficult to manage. To start, it is important to separate the facts from the myths. This is where seeking support from healthcare professionals comes in.

A diabetes educator or a registered dietitian can help you understand the science behind managing your condition and separate the truth from the fiction. They can guide you in developing a healthy lifestyle that works for you, including meal planning, exercise, and medication management.

Support a Diabetes Charity or Organization

Another great way to seek support is to become involved with a diabetes charity or organization. These groups offer a wealth of information and resources for people living with diabetes, as well as opportunities to connect with others who are going through the same experiences.

You can participate in events, join support groups, and get involved in advocacy efforts to help raise awareness of the condition and its impact.

Not only will you be helping others, but you will also find encouragement and comfort in being part of a community that understands your experiences.

Find a Hobby that is Not Diabetes Related

Finding a hobby or activity that you love is a great way to relieve stress and take your mind off diabetes. This can be anything from gardening to painting to playing an instrument. The key is to find something that you enjoy and that isn't tied to your diabetes management.

Not only will you feel happier, but you'll also find that taking time for yourself can help you manage your diabetes better in the long run.

Open and Honest Communication

Seeking support from loved ones is crucial. They can offer emotional support, but it's important to communicate your needs effectively. Don't be afraid to let them know what you need from them, but also be an active listener in return.

Be willing to have open and honest conversations about how diabetes is affecting you and your relationship with them. By doing so, you can build a stronger support network that will help you manage your diabetes and feel more confident in your daily life.

THE ROLE OF STRESS AND ANXIETY IN BLOOD SUGAR CONTROL

When you're stressed or anxious, your body goes into fight-or-flight mode. This means that it releases hormones like cortisol, adrenaline, and glucagon that can increase your blood sugar levels. In people without diabetes, this isn't usually a problem—their bodies produce enough insulin to bring their blood sugar back down to normal levels.

But if you have type 2 diabetes, your body may not be able to produce enough insulin or use it effectively, which can lead to a dangerous spike in blood sugar.

It's not just acute stress that can impact your blood sugar, either. Chronic stress and anxiety can also take a toll on your diabetes management. When you're in a constant state of stress, your body is constantly releasing those blood sugar-raising hormones.

Over time, this can cause insulin resistance, meaning that your cells become less responsive to the insulin that your body does produce. This can lead to higher and higher blood sugar levels, making it more difficult to manage your diabetes.

So, what can you do to lower the impact of stress and anxiety on your blood sugar? The first step is recognizing when you're experiencing these emotions and taking steps to manage them. This could mean practicing relaxation techniques like deep breathing, meditation, or yoga, talking to a therapist or counselor, or even just taking a walk outside. Experiment with different strategies and find what works best for you.

Another important step is staying consistent with the other aspects of your diabetes management. When you're stressed or anxious, it can be easy to let things like exercise, healthy eating, and medication management fall by the wayside.

But sticking to your routine as much as possible can help keep your blood sugar levels steady and make it easier to manage the effects of stress and anxiety.

HOW TO PRIORITIZE SELF-CARE AND MENTAL HEALTH IN DIABETES MANAGEMENT

Remember that managing your diabetes and taking care of your mental health should be your top priority. Many people with diabetes tend to put others first, but it's important to remember that self-care comes first. Taking time for yourself is not selfish; instead, it helps you take better care of your loved ones and your health.

Make a list of things that you enjoy doing and set aside time to do them. It could be anything from reading a book, taking a walk, or even watching a movie. Any activity that brings you joy and reduces stress should be at the top of your list.

Managing diabetes is more than just taking medication and keeping your blood sugar levels under control. It's also about prioritizing your mental health and self-care. By practicing mindful eating, connecting with loved ones, prioritizing sleep, and taking other steps, you can make yourself a priority and keep your diabetes symptoms in check.

Managing your mental health and emotional well-being with diabetes takes time, effort, and dedication. But with the right strategies and support, it's possible to live a life of balance and confidence.

One key step in this process is to assess all the options for treating and managing your type 2 diabetes. This will empower you to advocate for the specific treatment you need. Plus, being well-informed helps you show your healthcare providers that you are actively taking charge of your health to the best of your ability.

Finally, don't be afraid to reach out for help if you need it. Managing diabetes is tough, and dealing with the additional stress and anxiety that comes with it can make it even tougher. But you don't have to go it alone. I hope that's something you now recognize after reading this chapter.

At the end of the day, remember to acknowledge and manage your emotions, take care of your physical health, connect with others who understand, shift your perspective, and celebrate your successes.

In the next chapter, I'll give you a little more insight on how you can use that "fierce" attitude to advocate for your own health and wellbeing. Let's take a look!

10

ADVOCATING FOR YOUR HEALTH WITH TYPE 2 DIABETES

"Empowering people with diabetes helps them make informed choices."

— MARY MACKINNON

Advocating for your health means taking an active role in your care. It means speaking up when you have questions or concerns, being prepared for doctors' visits, and staying informed about the latest research and treatments.

By advocating for your health, you can make sure that you receive the care and support you need to manage your condition effectively.

That said, being an advocate for yourself isn't always easy. You need to be able to speak up when you have concerns and to ask questions when you're curious—even if you think your questions might be "stupid."

As they told you in grade school, there's no such thing as a stupid question—and that's especially true when it comes to managing your type 2 diabetes.

Here are some tips to help you become your own best spokesperson and advocate.

WHY IT'S IMPORTANT TO BE AN ACTIVE PARTICIPANT IN HEALTHCARE DECISIONS

As a diabetic, you are your own advocate when it comes to your health. Being an active participant in your healthcare is crucial to ensure you receive the best possible treatment and care.

Not only will your healthcare providers better understand your unique medical history and needs, but you'll be able to make decisions based on your personal preferences and values while managing a chronic condition like diabetes.

Active participation also helps you build a collaborative relationship with your healthcare team, which leads to better care and improved outcomes.

WHAT TO CONSIDER WHEN COMMUNICATING WITH HEALTHCARE PROFESSIONALS

Effective communication with your healthcare team is key to ensuring that you receive the best care possible.

It is important to be open and honest about your medical history, symptoms, and concerns. You should also take the initiative to ask questions about your diabetes care and treatment and discuss your options.

Keep a list of any questions or concerns you have and bring them with you to appointments. This helps ensure that your healthcare provider addresses all your concerns and questions.

Bring any information from other providers such as labs, notes, and medication lists or changes. This helps communication between specialties, so everyone has an accurate picture of what is going on.

Remember, your healthcare team is there to help, and the more you communicate, the better they can assist you.

Questions to ask your healthcare provider.

Before starting any medication for diabetes, it's essential to have an open and thorough conversation with your healthcare provider to ensure the chosen medication is both safe and effective for your specific needs. To help guide your discussion, here are ten important questions you should consider asking your doctor or pharmacist:

1. What is the primary function of this medication?

Ask your healthcare provider about the intended purpose of the medication, how it works, and the expected benefits for your blood sugar management.

2. How and when should I take this medication?

Inquire about the appropriate dosage, timing, and whether the medication should be taken with or without food. This information is crucial to ensure proper absorption and effectiveness.

3. Can I take this medication with other drugs?

Discuss potential interactions with other medications you are currently taking and learn about any warning signs of adverse drug interactions.

4. Are there side effects or interactions with food or supplements?

Understand the potential side effects and any interactions with specific foods, beverages, or dietary supplements that could affect the medication's effectiveness or safety.

5. How long will it take before the medication begins to work?

Ask your healthcare provider about the expected time frame for the medication to start showing its effects on your diabetes.

6. How can I determine if the medication is working, and how frequently should I monitor my blood glucose?

Learn how to evaluate the effectiveness of your medication and the recommended frequency for blood sugar monitoring.

7. Are there any lifestyle changes I should make while taking this medication?

Discuss any recommended adjustments to your diet, exercise routine, or other lifestyle factors that may complement your high blood sugar treatment plan.

8. What precautions should I take while on this medication?

Understand any specific precautions you should be aware of while taking the medication, such as avoiding activities, foods, or beverages.

9. What should I do if I miss a dose or accidentally take too much medication?

Learn the appropriate steps to take in case you miss a dose or accidentally take more medication than prescribed.

10. When should I schedule a follow-up appointment to assess my blood sugar and evaluate the medication's effectiveness?

Determine the optimal time for a follow-up appointment to review your blood sugar levels and discuss the medication's effectiveness with your healthcare provider.

By asking these vital questions and staying informed about your medication and its potential interactions, you can better manage your high blood sugar and reduce the risk of complications. Remember, active involvement in your treatment plan and open communication with your healthcare team is key to achieving optimal blood sugar control and improving your overall health.

PATIENT RIGHTS AS A DIABETIC

It is essential to understand what your rights are, so you can exercise them, and take control of your health.

To start with, as a diabetic, you have the right to access medical care without discrimination. This means that doctors cannot refuse to see you or provide adequate care based on your diabetes. It also means that insurance companies cannot deny you coverage or charge you higher premiums because of your condition.

Diabetes management requires medication and regular testing, and you have the right to both. Your healthcare provider should help you find affordable medication and provide you with the necessary test supplies. If you are having trouble getting access to medication, seek out resources, like assistance programs or patient advocacy groups. Often manufacturers offer assistance programs or coupons for meters and sometimes testing supplies. Hospitals and clinics often have case workers that can help you get affordable supplies.

Also, you have the right to make decisions about your care, including which physician you see, what medications you take, and what treatments you undergo. Do not be afraid to speak up and ask questions during your appointments. Your healthcare providers should collaborate with you to develop a care plan that suits your needs.

THE ROLE OF TECHNOLOGY IN DIABETES MANAGEMENT

Living with diabetes can be tough. It takes a lot of hard work and dedication to maintain good blood sugar levels, and even then, it can still be a challenge. But here is some good news, technology is making diabetes management easier than ever before.

From blood glucose monitors to insulin pumps, there is a range of new devices available that can help you better control your blood sugar levels. And it is not just about the hardware—software and apps are also playing a role in diabetes management.

Let us start with blood glucose monitors. For many people with diabetes, monitoring blood sugar levels is a daily task. But traditional monitors can be painful and difficult to use. Today, there are better options available. Some monitors now offer pain-free testing, while others connect to an app so you can monitor your levels on your phone. There are even monitors that can automatically share your results with your doctor, giving them a better understanding of your overall health.

Another device that is gaining popularity is the smart insulin pen. This is a device that tracks your insulin doses and sends the information to your smartphone. It can also remind you when it is time for your next dose, helping you stay on top of your medication. For people who use insulin regularly, this could be a real game-changer.

Then there are insulin pumps. These devices make it easier to manage insulin therapy, as they deliver insulin automatically throughout the day. They can also be adjusted to match your activity levels and food intake, giving you more control over your blood sugar levels.

And like many other devices, they can be used in conjunction with an app to help you track your progress.

Technology is not just about hardware, though. There are also apps and software that can help with diabetes management.

For example, there are apps that can track what you eat and suggest healthy alternatives, helping you make better food choices. Others can remind you to take medication, monitor your blood glucose levels, or even offer support from other people with diabetes.

SELF-ADVOCACY FOR BETTER HEALTH OUTCOMES

Self-advocacy is also important when it comes to diabetes management. This means taking an active role in your own health and making sure you have the tools and resources you need to manage your condition. Technology can help with this, but it's important to be informed and to understand what's available.

Self-advocacy in a healthcare setting refers to the practice of patients or individuals taking an active and informed role in advocating for their own healthcare needs, preferences, and rights. It involves asserting one's interests, asking questions, and making decisions regarding their medical care, treatment options, and overall well-being. Self-advocacy is essential in empowering patients to:

1. Communicate Effectively: Express their concerns, symptoms, and medical history clearly to healthcare providers, ensuring accurate and comprehensive information is available for diagnosis and treatment.

2. Make Informed Decisions: Gather information about their medical condition, treatment options, potential risks, and benefits, enabling them to make informed decisions in collaboration with healthcare professionals.
3. Ask Questions: Seek clarification, ask questions, and request additional information about their diagnosis, treatment plan, and medications to ensure they understand and are comfortable with the proposed care.
4. Assert Preferences: Share their preferences and values regarding treatment approaches, pain management, and end-of-life care, allowing healthcare providers to tailor care to individual needs.
5. Advocate for Rights: Be aware of their legal and ethical rights as patients, including the right to informed consent, confidentiality, and access to medical records, and assert these rights when necessary.
6. Monitor Care: Keep track of their healthcare journey, including appointments, medications, and symptoms, to help identify any issues or discrepancies in their care.
7. Seek Second Opinions: If uncertain or dissatisfied with a diagnosis or treatment plan, patients can seek second opinions from other healthcare professionals to ensure the best possible care.

8. Address Concerns: Speak up if they experience any discomfort, side effects, or complications related to their treatment, ensuring timely interventions and adjustments.
9. Collaborate with Care Team: Work collaboratively with healthcare providers, nurses, and other members of the care team to achieve the best possible health outcomes.

Overall, self-advocacy in healthcare empowers individuals to actively participate in their healthcare decision-making process, promote their own well-being, and ensure that their medical care aligns with their values and preferences. It is particularly important in today's patient-centered healthcare systems, where shared decision-making and patient engagement are valued practices.

SPECIAL CONSIDERATIONS FOR DIABETES MANAGEMENT

Diabetes management differs depending on the demographic. Here are a few general guidelines for diabetes management across age groups.

Children

Managing diabetes in children can be challenging because they may not fully understand the disease and its impact on their daily lives. Plus, children often have difficulty adhering to strict diet and medication schedules.

As a result, caretakers must be particularly vigilant about monitoring blood sugar levels and ensuring children with diabetes receive appropriate support and education.

Adolescents

Adolescence is a time of significant physical and emotional changes, which can make diabetes management even more challenging. Adolescents with diabetes often struggle with self-care and maintaining healthy habits amidst peer pressure and other distractions.

One way to engage adolescents with diabetes in their care is to incorporate technology into their self-management routine.

For example, some teens may benefit from using diabetes management apps and wearable devices to track their blood sugar levels, physical activity, and medication adherence.

Elderly

Diabetes management in the elderly is often complicated by other health conditions and medications, which can interfere with blood sugar control. In addition, elderly patients may have difficulty adhering to strict dietary and exercise guidelines due to decreased mobility and cognitive function.

One way to support elderly patients with diabetes is to establish a strong care team that includes family members, healthcare providers, and pharmacists. It's also essential to customize treatment plans based on individual needs and preferences.

Because many elderly patients with diabetes have had the condition for many years, it's also important to recognize that your treatment and management of diabetes might change as you age.

Just take the example of Bob Krause, who died at the age of 90 due to complications unrelated to diabetes. Bob spent more than 85 years of his life with diabetes. He went down in history as the first American to live with diabetes for 85 years, and he witnessed remarkable changes as treatments for diabetes evolve over time.

Bob outlived the life expectancy of a normal healthy person born in 1921. -While he always knew he had to deal with his diabetes, he also recognized that it's just a part of his life and it doesn't need to control his life.

Perspective is everything, Bob is excellent proof of this.

CONCLUSION

Perspective is everything. That's something I said in the last chapter, and it's something I've reiterated continuously throughout this book.

While type 2 diabetes isn't necessarily something that's "fun" or "cool" to live with, the reality is that you can't change the diagnosis. The only thing you can change is your mindset.

Managing type 2 diabetes can be a daunting task, but it doesn't have to be. Often, we view diabetes as an enemy, and the thought of having to control what we eat, constantly monitor our blood sugar levels, and take medication can take a toll on us physically and mentally.

But what if we shift our perspective and look at it as a chance to take charge of our health?

Through the right mindset and perspective, we can turn what may seem like a burden into an opportunity to improve our overall well-being.

While it may be overwhelming to think about all the things that you cannot eat or do as a person living with type 2 diabetes, it's essential to focus on what you can control.

Take time to plan and prepare meals that are healthy and enjoyable at the same time. Engage in physical activities that bring you joy, and do not be afraid to try new things. Every person is different, and so is their experience with managing type 2 diabetes. Focus on finding what works best for you and incorporating it into your lifestyle.

Knowledge is power, and when it comes to managing type 2 diabetes, understanding the condition is crucial. Educate yourself on what type 2 diabetes is, the medication you are taking, and how to monitor your blood sugar levels.

The more you know, the more equipped you will be to make informed decisions and manage the condition effectively.

Hopefully, you now know the skills, techniques, and basic information you need to feel as though you can take charge of your type 2 diabetes. We have covered all the basics in this book so that you can control every aspect of your type 2 diabetes, including your:

- Mental health and emotional wellbeing
- Suitable lifestyle modifications

- Medications and the ability to adhere to them as prescribed
- Accountability, adherence, and self-advocacy for your own health

When we change the way we think about and view things, we empower ourselves to make better decisions and take control of our health.

Just take the example of Nan Hilton.

Nan was diagnosed with type 2 diabetes in 2006 at just 23 years old.

She took medications and insulin for years. When she became pregnant in 2010, she knew something needed to change. Her pregnancy was considered high-risk due to her diabetes, and during her pregnancy, she developed severe diabetic retinopathy that caused vision loss and required complicated, invasive surgery.

Her life changed dramatically due to her diabetes, to a debilitating point. After giving birth, she knew it was time for a major overhaul.

Nan made some basic lifestyle modifications (such as incorporating aerobic activity and changing her diet) that resulted in a 90-pound weight loss. Today, Nan no longer relies on diabetes medications. She leans on her family for support and relies on them to continue to provide her with the motivation she needs to stay on track.

You can do this, too.

Always remember, you are not alone. Millions of people are managing their type 2 diabetes and thriving. And with the right tools and support, you can too.

It has been a pleasure to walk you through everything you need to know about type 2 diabetes. I am hoping that this book has given you the confidence you need to take back control of your health and well-being.

If you enjoyed this book, please leave me a review. This will help other people like yourself find the book and access the information *they* need to take charge of their type 2 diabetes, too. As I have said repeatedly, knowledge is power. So please take the time to pay it forward and help others access this knowledge, too.

As Dale Evans famously said, "Life is not over because you have diabetes. Make the most of what you have."

Hopefully, this book has given you everything you need to move forward—and to live a healthy, prosperous life with type 2 diabetes.

GLOSSARY

Adiposity- body fat

Anabolic steroids- synthetic (man-made) versions of testosterone

Blood lipid levels- a panel of blood tests used to find abnormalities in lipids such as cholesterol and triglycerides

Blood Sugar- the concentration of glucose in the blood

Cataracts- a medical condition in which the lens of the eye becomes progressively opaque resulting in blurred vision

Cholesterol- a compound found in cell membranes and precursor to steroid compounds

Cognitive Function- brain functions (attention, memory, and processing speed)

Cortisol- A steroid hormone that your adrenal glands produce and release

Diabetic coma- severely high or low glucose levels can cause unresponsiveness

Emaciation- extreme loss of muscle and fat under the skin from malnutrition

Epigenetic- the study of how your behaviors and environment can cause changes that affect the way your genes work

Glaucoma- nerve damage in the eye from high eye pressure causing blindness

Glucagon- a hormone formed in the pancreas which promotes the breakdown of glycogen to glucose in the liver

Glucose- a simple sugar which is an important energy source and a component in carbohydrates

Glucose Meters- a device for measuring the concentration of glucose in the blood

Glycemic control- a medical term referring to the typical levels of blood sugar (glucose) in a person with diabetes mellitus.

Glycemic Index- a system that ranks foods on a scale from 1 to 100 based on their effect on blood sugar levels

HbA1c (A1c)- Hemoglobin A1C measures the amount of blood sugar (glucose) attached to your hemoglobin.

HDL- high-density lipoprotein is a type of cholesterol, sometimes called "good" cholesterol, which absorbs cholesterol in the blood and carries it back to the liver

Hyperglycemia- an excess of glucose in the bloodstream

Hypoglycemia- deficiency of glucose in the bloodstream

Insulin- a hormone produced in the pancreas which regulates the amount of glucose in the blood

Insulin Pump- An insulin pump is a medical device used for the administration of insulin in the treatment of diabetes

Insulin Resistance- an impaired response of the body to insulin resulting in elevated levels of glucose in the blood

Ketoacidosis- "Diabetic ketoacidosis" is a serious complication where the body produces excess blood acids (ketones)

Ketones- an organic compound that the liver produces when it breaks down fats

Metabolic Dysfunction- when something is wrong with the body's metabolism

Metabolic Syndrome- multiple abnormalities associated with the development of cardiovascular disease and type 2 diabetes

Net carbs- the total amount of fully digestible carbohydrates contained within a product or meal

Neuropathy- disease or dysfunction of one or more peripheral nerves typically causing numbness and weakness

Nocturnal Hypoglycemia- low blood sugar levels at night in a person who has diabetes

Obesity- the state or condition of being very fat or overweight

Prediabetes- impaired glucose tolerance

Retinopathy- a complication of diabetes that affects the eyes damaging blood vessels and leading to vision loss

Steroids- organic compounds in the body that makeup hormones

Triglycerides- the main constituents of natural fats and oils, high concentrations in the blood indicate an elevated risk of stroke

REFERENCES

Alcohol and diabetes. (n.d.). ADA. https://diabetes.org/healthy-living/medication-treatments/alcohol-diabetes

Are there any safety considerations for people with diabetes when they exercise? (n.d.). ViMax Media. Retrieved June 15, 2023, from http://erlr.org/generic/articles/diabetic-smart/are-there-any-safety-considerations-for-people-with-diabetes-when-they-exercise/

Assid, P. (2021). Diabetes and shortness of breath: What's the cause? *Verywell Health*. https://www.verywellhealth.com/diabetes-and-shortness-of-breath-5114863

Blood glucose. (n.d.). MedlinePlus. https://medlineplus.gov/bloodsugar.html

Blood glucose and insulin at work. (n.d.). ADA. https://diabetes.org/tools-support/diabetes-prevention/high-blood-sugar

Blood sugar testing: Why, when, and how. (2022). Mayo Clinic. https://www.mayoclinic.org/diseases-conditions/diabetes/in-depth/blood-sugar/art-20046628

BNF is only available in the UK. (n.d.). NICE. https://bnf.nice.org.uk/treatment-summaries/hypoglycaemia/

Budson, A. E. (2021). What's the relationship between diabetes and dementia? *Harvard Health*. https://www.health.harvard.edu/blog/whats-the-relationship-between-diabetes-and-dementia-202107122546

Callahan, A. (2018). 7 medications that may affect blood sugar control in diabetes. *EverydayHealth*. https://www.everydayhealth.com/type-2-diabetes/treatment/medications-may-affect-blood-sugar-control-diabetes/

Carbohydrates: How carbs fit into a healthy diet. (2022). Mayo Clinic. https://www.mayoclinic.org/healthy-lifestyle/nutrition-and-healthy-eating/in-depth/carbohydrates/art-20045705

Carbohydrates, proteins, fats, and blood sugar. (n.d.). HealthLink BC. https://www.healthlinkbc.ca/healthy-eating-physical-activity/food-and-nutrition/nutrients/carbohydrate-proteins-fats-and-blood

Care, D. (2018). 10 tips for effective communication with your doctor.

Diabetes Care Community. https://www.diabetescarecommunity.ca/living-well-with-diabetes-articles/10-tips-for-effective-communication-with-your-doctor/

CDC. (2018). All about your A1C. *Centers for Disease Control and Prevention.* https://www.cdc.gov/diabetes/managing/managing-blood-sugar/a1c.html

CDC. (2021). Make the connection. *Centers for Disease Control and Prevention.* https://www.cdc.gov/diabetes/managing/diabetes-kidney-disease.html

CDC. (2022a). Diabetes symptoms. *Centers for Disease Control and Prevention.* https://www.cdc.gov/diabetes/basics/symptoms.html

CDC. (2022b). Diabetes risk factors. *Centers for Disease Control and Prevention.* https://www.cdc.gov/diabetes/basics/risk-factors.html

CDC. (2022c). 10 tips for coping with diabetes distress. *Centers for Disease Control and Prevention.* https://www.cdc.gov/diabetes/managing/diabetes-distress/ten-tips-coping-diabetes-distress.html

CDC. (2022d). Sleep for a good cause. *Centers for Disease Control and Prevention.* https://www.cdc.gov/diabetes/library/features/diabetes-sleep.html

CDC. (2022e). What causes type 2 diabetes. *Centers for Disease Control and Prevention.* https://www.cdc.gov/diabetes/library/features/diabetes-causes.html

CDC. (2023a). Meal planning. *Centers for Disease Control and Prevention.* https://www.cdc.gov/diabetes/managing/eat-well/meal-plan-method.html

CDC. (2023b). Diabetes and mental health. *Centers for Disease Control and Prevention.* https://www.cdc.gov/diabetes/managing/mental-health.html

Chapple, Bridget. (n.d.). Stress and diabetes. *Diabetes UK.* https://www.diabetes.org.uk/guide-to-diabetes/emotions/stress

Cervoni, B. (2021). Are you more likely to get diabetes if it runs in your family? *Verywell Health.* https://www.verywellhealth.com/is-diabetes-genetic-5112506

Cherney, K. (2018). A complete list of diabetes medications. *Healthline Media.* https://www.healthline.com/health/diabetes/medications-list#type-1-diabetes

Chesak, J. (2020). What does insulin cost and what's behind the skyrocketing prices? *Verywell Health.* https://www.verywellhealth.com/insulin-prices-how-much-does-insulin-cost-and-why-5081872

Cervoni, Barbie. (2023). Could your diabetes medication stop working? *Verywell Health.* https://www.verywellhealth.com/diabetes-medication-not-working-6822997

Dening, J. (2022). What's the connection between diabetes and wound healing? *Healthline Media.* https://www.healthline.com/health/diabetes/diabetes-and-wound-healing

Devices & technology. (n.d.). ADA. https://diabetes.org/tools-support/devices-technology

Diabetes success stories. (2018). UMass Chan Medical School. https://www.umassmed.edu/dcoe/diabetes-care/success-stories/

Diabetes: 12 warning signs that appear on your skin. (n.d.). https://www.aad.org/public/diseases/a-z/diabetes-warning-signs

Diabetes and alcohol. (n.d.). WebMD. https://www.webmd.com/diabetes/guide/drinking-alcohol

Diabetes and blood sugar testing. (n.d.). WebMD. https://www.webmd.com/diabetes/home-blood-glucose-testing

Diabetes and cancer. (n.d.). ADA. https://diabetes.org/tools-support/diabetes-prevention/diabetes-and-cancer

Diabetes and dementia risk: Another good reason to keep blood sugar in check. (2021). Heart.org. https://www.heart.org/en/news/2021/07/21/diabetes-and-dementia-risk-another-good-reason-to-keep-blood-sugar-in-check

Diabetes and dietary supplements. (n.d.-). WebMD. https://www.webmd.com/diabetes/diabetes-dietary-supplements

Diabetes and dietary supplements. (n.d.). NCCIH. https://www.nccih.nih.gov/health/diabetes-and-dietary-supplements

Diabetes and exercise–Diabetes Stories. (n.d.). Diabetes Stories.https://diabetesstories.com/category/diabetes-and-exercise/

Diabetes and exercise: When to monitor your blood sugar. (2022). Mayo Clinic. https://www.mayoclinic.org/diseases-conditions/diabetes/in-depth/diabetes-and-exercise/art-20045697

Diabetes and Family History: How Much Risk is Genetic? (n.d.). YourDiabetesInfo.Org. https://yourdiabetesinfo.org/familyhistory/

Diabetes care and the adolescent population: Navigating the transition of roles and

responsibilities. (2022). NIDDK - National Institute of Diabetes and Digestive and Kidney Diseases. https://www.niddk.nih.gov/health-information/professionals/diabetes-discoveries-practice/managing-diabetes-transition

Diabetes diet: Create your healthy-eating plan. (2023). Mayo Clinic. https://www.mayoclinic.org/diseases-conditions/diabetes/in-depth/diabetes-diet/art-20044295

Diabetes management: How lifestyle, daily routine affects blood sugar. (2022). Mayo Clinic. https://www.mayoclinic.org/diseases-conditions/diabetes/in-depth/diabetes-management/art-20047963

Diabetes risk factors. (2018). Www.Heart.Org. https://www.heart.org/en/health-topics/diabetes/understand-your-risk-for-diabetes

Diabetes statistics. (2023). NIDDK: National Institute of Diabetes and Digestive and Kidney Diseases. https://www.niddk.nih.gov/health-information/health-statistics/diabetes-statistics

Diabetes: Stress & depression. Cleveland Clinic. (n.d.). https://my.clevelandclinic.org/health/articles/14891-diabetes-stress--depression

Diabetes treatment: Medications for type 2 diabetes. (2022). Mayo Clinic. https://www.mayoclinic.org/diseases-conditions/type-2-diabetes/in-depth/diabetes-treatment/art-20051004

Diabetes: What you need to know as you age. (2023). Johns Hopkins Medicine. https://www.hopkinsmedicine.org/health/conditions-and-diseases/diabetes/diabetes-what-you-need-to-know-as-you-age

Diabetic calorie counting chart. (2017). Diabetestalk.Net. https://diabetestalk.net/blood-sugar/diabetic-calorie-counting-chart

Diabetic nephropathy (kidney disease)— Symptoms and causes. (2021). Mayo Clinic. https://www.mayoclinic.org/diseases-conditions/diabetic-nephropathy/symptoms-causes/syc-20354556

Diabetic neuropathy. (2020). Johns Hopkins Medicine. https://www.hopkinsmedicine.org/health/conditions-and-diseases/diabetes/diabetic-neuropathy-nerve-problems

Diabetic neuropathy— Symptoms and causes. (2022). Mayo Clinic. https://www.mayoclinic.org/diseases-conditions/diabetic-neuropathy/symptoms-causes/syc-20371580

Diabetic retinopathy—Symptoms and causes. (2023). Mayo Clinic. https://www.mayoclinic.org/diseases-conditions/diabetic-retinopathy/symptoms-causes/syc-20371611

Do I need to change my type 2 diabetes medication? (n.d.). WebMD. https://www.webmd.com/diabetes/change-type-2-diabetes-meds

Drugs vs. lifestyle for preventing diabetes. (2016). NutritionFacts.Org. https://nutritionfacts.org/2016/03/08/drugs-vs-lifestyle-for-preventing-diabetes/

Doskicz, J. (2018). These 9 drugs may raise your blood sugar. *GoodRx.* https://www.goodrx.com/conditions/diabetes/drugs-that-raise-blood-sugar

Erectile dysfunction and diabetes: Take control today. (2023). Mayo Clinic. https://www.mayoclinic.org/diseases-conditions/erectile-dysfunction/in-depth/erectile-dysfunction/art-20043927

Exercise and diabetes. (2019). The Johns Hopkins Patient Guide to Diabetes. https://hopkinsdiabetesinfo.org/exercise-and-diabetes/

Exercise can raise blood glucose (blood sugar). (n.d.). ADA. https://diabetes.org/healthy-living/fitness/why-does-exercise-sometimes-raise-blood-sugar

Exercising safely with diabetes. (2016). Harvard Health. https://www.health.harvard.edu/diseases-and-conditions/exercising-safely-with-diabetes

Fallabel, C. (2022). Know your hospital rights as a person with diabetes. *Diabetes Daily.* https://www.diabetesdaily.com/learn-about-diabetes/living-with-diabetes/navigating-the-healthcare-system-with-diabetes/know-your-hospital-rights-as-a-person-with-diabetes/

Family health history and diabetes. (2023). CDC. https://www.cdc.gov/genomics/famhistory/famhist_diabetes.htm

The link between diabetes and sexual dysfunction. (2020). Cleveland Clinic. https://health.clevelandclinic.org/the-link-between-diabetes-and-sexual-dysfunction/

Fletcher, J. (2019). A list of healthier foods for people with diabetes, and foods to limit or avoid. *Medical News Today.* https://www.medicalnewstoday.com/articles/317355

Gasnick, K. (2023). Addressing sedentary lifestyle with type 2 diabetes. *Verywell Health.* https://www.verywellhealth.com/addressing-sedentary-lifestyle-with-type-2-diabetes-6606484

Genetics of diabetes. (n.d.). ADA. https://diabetes.org/diabetes/genetics-diabetes

Glucose Metabolism—An overview. (n.d.). ScienceDirect Topics. https://www.sciencedirect.com/topics/medicine-and-dentistry/glucose-metabolism

Gourmet, D. (2017). Best diabetes websites – hand-picked list. *Diabetic*

Gourmet Magazine. https://diabeticgourmet.com/articles/best-diabetes-websites-hand-picked-list

Gray, A., & Threlkeld, R. J. (2019). Nutritional recommendations for individuals with diabetes. *NCBI Bookshelf.* https://www.ncbi.nlm.nih.gov/books/NBK279012/

Gunnars, K. (2021). Carbohydrates: Whole vs. refined—here's the difference. *Healthline Media.* https://www.healthline.com/nutrition/good-carbs-bad-carbs

Halvorson, M., Yasuda, P., Carpenter, S., & Kaiserman, K. (2005). Unique challenges for pediatric patients with diabetes. *Diabetes Spectrum, 18*(3), 167–173. https://doi.org/10.2337/diaspect.18.3.167

Hazlegreaves, S. (2019). Technology and diabetes: How can innovation address the mounting challenge? *Open Access Government.* https://www.openaccessgovernment.org/technology-diabetes-challenge/59130/

Health checks for people with diabetes. (n.d.). ADA. https://diabetes.org/diabetes/newly-diagnosed/health-checks-people-with-diabetes

Herndon, J. (2021). What to know about steroid-induced diabetes. *Healthline Media.* https://www.healthline.com/health/diabetes/steroid-induced-diabetes

Hoskins, M. (2022). Helping you understand 'normal' blood sugar levels. *Healthline Media.* https://www.healthline.com/health/diabetes/normal-blood-sugar-level#target-glucose-goals

How can you support someone with diabetes in a nonjudgmental way? (2021b). *Verywell Health.* https://www.verywellhealth.com/supporting-someone-with-diabetes-5206667

How diabetes affects employment and daily work. (2019). dQ&A. https://d-qa.com/how-diabetes-affects-employment-and-daily-work/

How secreted insulin works in your body. (n.d.). WebMD. https://www.webmd.com/diabetes/insulin-explained

How sleep affects blood sugar. (n.d.). WebMD. https://www.webmd.com/diabetes/sleep-affects-blood-sugar

How to prioritize self-care and your mental health. (n.d.). Nivati. https://www.nivati.com/blog/how-to-prioritize-self-care-and-your-mental-health

Hwang, K. O. (2020). Type 2 diabetes: A doctor's guide to a good appointment. *Healthline Media.* https://www.healthline.com/health/type-2-diabetes/guide-to-appointment#What-to-share-with-your-doctor

Importance of medication adherence in diabetes. (2018). Apollo Sugar Clinics. https://apollosugar.com/world-of-diabetes/diabetes-management/importance-of-medication-adherence-in-diabetes/

Injury-free exercise tips. (n.d.). ADA. https://diabetes.org/healthy-living/fitness/getting-started-safely/injury-free-exercise-11-quick-safety-tips

Inspirational stories. (2019). Know Diabetes by Heart. https://www.knowdiabetesbyheart.org/resources/inspiring-stories/

Insulin. (n.d.). Cleveland Clinic. https://my.clevelandclinic.org/health/articles/22601-insulin

Insulin resistance. (n.d.). WebMD. https://www.webmd.com/diabetes/insulin-resistance-syndrome

1 in 10 people are living with diabetes. International Diabetes Federation (IDF) https://www.idf.org/52-about-diabetes/43-rights-and-responsibilities.html

Is diabetes a disability? Understanding your rights and benefits. (2023). Disability Works, https://disabilityworks.org/is-diabetes-a-disability-understanding-your-rights-and-benefits/

Janaway, D. B. (2017). Understanding diabetes jargon. *Patient.* https://patient.info/news-and-features/understanding-diabetes-jargon

Jaspan, R. (2022). 1-Week meal plan & recipe prep for pre-diabetes. *Verywell Fit.* https://www.verywellfit.com/1-week-pre-diabetic-meal-plan-ideas-recipes-and-prep-6504170

Kalra, S., Jena, B. N., & Yeravdekar, R. (2018). Emotional and psychological needs of people with diabetes. *Indian Journal of Endocrinology and Metabolism, 22*(5). https://doi.org/10.4103/ijem.IJEM_579_17

Lachtrupp, E. (2021). Diabetes meal plan for beginners. *EatingWell.* https://www.eatingwell.com/article/7886108/diabetes-meal-plan-for-beginners/

Lando, H. M., & Ragone, M. (2001). Case study: A 68-year-old man with diabetes and peripheral neuropathy. *Clinical Diabetes, 19*(3), 122–123. https://doi.org/10.2337/diaclin.19.3.122

Landry, J. (2023, February 17). *72+ best diabetes quotes and sayings for inspiration (2023).* Respiratory Therapy Zone. https://www.respiratorytherapyzone.com/diabetes-quotes/

Lee, A. M. I. (2019). Self-Advocacy: What it is and why it's important. *Understood.* https://www.understood.org/en/articles/the-importance-of-self-advocacy

Lee, A. R. (2022). How do insulin and blood sugar work in diabetes? *Verywell Health*. https://www.verywellhealth.com/insulin-vs-blood-sugar-how-to-manage-type-2-diabetes-6740387

Lee, A. R. (2023). Drugs that raise blood sugar and can complicate diabetes. *Verywell Health*. https://www.verywellhealth.com/list-of-drugs-that-raise-blood-sugar-6542910

Leung, E., Wongrakpanich, S., & Munshi, M. N. (2018). Diabetes management in the elderly. *Diabetes Spectrum, 31*(3), 245–253. https://doi.org/10.2337/ds18-0033

Lifestyle changes can prevent or delay diabetes. (2022). Verywell Health. https://www.verywellhealth.com/lifestyle-changes-for-diabetes-prevention-6543350

Lifestyle vs. Medication: Which is More Powerful for Maintaining a Healthy Weight? (2016). Ask The Scientists. https://askthescientists.com/lifestyle-improvements-effective-medications-reducing-diabetes-risk/

Living healthy with diabetes. (2018). Www.Heart.Org. https://www.heart.org/en/health-topics/diabetes/prevention--treatment-of-diabetes/living-healthy-with-diabetes

Living my best life with type 2 diabetes. (2020). WebMD. https://www.webmd.com/diabetes/diabetes-perspectives-21/type-2-everyday-life

Lodhia, H. (2023). The power of self-care: Prioritizing mental health in a busy world! *My Publication*. https://drhenalodhia.substack.com/p/the-power-of-self-care-prioritizing

Managing stress when you have diabetes. (n.d.). WebMD. https://www.webmd.com/diabetes/managing-stress

Marcin, A. (2018). *How are carbohydrates digested?* Healthline Media. https://www.healthline.com/health/carbohydrate-digestion#digestion-process

MBE, D. S. J. (2021). Why type 2 diabetes check-ups are so important. *Patient*. https://patient.info/news-and-features/why-you-should-go-for-regular-check-ups-if-you-have-type-2-diabetes

McCament-Mann, L. A. (n.d.). A New Class of Drugs for Diabetes. *National Capital Poison Center*. https://www.poison.org/articles/benefits-and-risks-new-diabetes-drugs-183

McCoy, K. (). The history of diabetes. *EverydayHealth.Com*. https://www.everydayhealth.com/diabetes/understanding/diabetes-mellitus-through-time.aspx

Meds that can spike your blood sugar. (n.d.). WebMD. https://www.webmd.com/diabetes/medicines-blood-sugar-spike

Meissner, M. (2021). How diabetes affects men vs. women. *Medical News Today.* https://www.medicalnewstoday.com/articles/diabetes-affects-men-women

Metabolic syndrome. (2021). Johns Hopkins Medicine. https://www.hopkinsmedicine.org/health/conditions-and-diseases/metabolic-syndrome

Metabolic syndrome—Symptoms and causes. (2021). Mayo Clinic. https://www.mayoclinic.org/diseases-conditions/metabolic-syndrome/symptoms-causes/syc-20351916

Muccioli, M. (2022). Are people with diabetes immunocompromised? *Diabetes Daily.* https://www.diabetesdaily.com/blog/author/mariamuccioli/

National Diabetes Statistics Report. (2022). CDC. https://www.cdc.gov/diabetes/data/statistics-report/index.html

National DPP Customer Service Center. (n.d.). https://nationaldppcsc.cdc.gov/s/article/CDC-2022-National-Diabetes-Statistics-Report

Nellis, P. (2021). Self-Advocacy leads to better health & well-being. *Occupational Therapy Services.* https://otservices.wustl.edu/self-advocacy-leads-to-better-health-well-being/

New technologies in diabetes care and management. (2023). NIDDK: National Institute of Diabetes and Digestive and Kidney Diseases. https://www.niddk.nih.gov/health-information/professionals/diabetes-discoveries-practice/new-technologies-in-diabetes-care-and-management

Normal fasting and postprandial blood glucose levels. (2018). Diabetestalk.Net. https://diabetestalk.net/blood-sugar/normal-fasting-and-postprandial-blood-glucose-levels

Oral and non-insulin medications. (2016). The Johns Hopkins Patient Guide to Diabetes. https://hopkinsdiabetesinfo.org/treatments/oral-medications/

Osborn, C. O. (2020). Type 1 and type 2 diabetes: What's the difference? *Healthline Media.* https://www.healthline.com/health/difference-between-type-1-and-type-2-diabetes

Pacheco, D. (2020a). Diabetes and sleep: Sleep disturbances & coping. *Sleep Foundation.* https://www.sleepfoundation.org/physical-health/lack-of-sleep-and-diabetes

Pacheco, D. (2020b). Sleep & glucose: How blood sugar can affect rest. *Sleep*

Foundation. https://www.sleepfoundation.org/physical-health/sleep-and-blood-glucose-levels

Pancreas. (n.d.). Cleveland Clinic. https://my.clevelandclinic.org/health/body/21743-pancreas

Panoff, L. (2022, November 28). Obesity and diabetes: Connection, risk, and management. *Verywell Health*. https://www.verywellhealth.com/obesity-and-diabetes-6823190

Patient stories. (). The Johns Hopkins Patient Guide to Diabetes. https://hopkinsdiabetesinfo.org/patient-stories/

Pon, E. du, Wildeboer, A. T., van Dooren, A. A., Bilo, H. J. G., Kleefstra, N., & van Dulmen, S. (2019). Active participation of patients with type 2 diabetes in consultations with their primary care practice nurses—What helps and what hinders: A qualitative study. *BMC Health Services Research, 19*(1), 1–11. https://doi.org/10.1186/s12913-019-4572-5

Poulson, B. (2021). Type 2 diabetes complications: Overview and more. *Verywell Health*. https://www.verywellhealth.com/type-2-diabetes-complications-5120942

Prevalence of Diagnosed Diabetes. (2022). CDC. https://www.cdc.gov/diabetes/data/statistics-report/diagnosed-diabetes.html

Price, C. (2013). A diabetes exercise success story. *ASweetLife*. https://asweetlife.org/a-diabetes-exercise-success-story/

Purdie, J. (2016). Stress: How it affects diabetes and how to decrease it. *Healthline Media*. https://www.healthline.com/health/diabetes-and-stress

Ries, J. (2020). 40% of people with type 2 diabetes initially avoid insulin therapy. *Healthline Media*. https://www.healthline.com/health-news/why-delaying-insulin-is-dangerous-in-the-long-run

Rowley, W. R., Bezold, C., Arikan, Y., Byrne, E., & Krohe, S. (2017). Diabetes 2030: Insights from yesterday, today, and future trends. *Population Health Management, 20*(1). https://doi.org/10.1089/pop.2015.0181

Sample menu for patients with diabetes. (n.d.). Sutter Health. https://www.sutterhealth.org/health/diabetes/diabetic-meal-plan

Seery, C. (2019). Diabetes real life stories. *Diabetes*. https://www.diabetes.co.uk/diabetes-real-life-stories.html

Shaikh, J. (2021). Why is diabetes increasing in the United States? MedicineNet. https://www.medicinenet.com/why_is_diabetes_increasing_in_the_united_stat/article.htm=

Singh, K. (2019a). Diabetes jargon, abbreviations, and terminology. *Diabetes.* https://www.diabetes.co.uk/diabetes-jargon.html

Singh, K. (2019b). Poor blood circulation - Causes, association with diabetes, treatment. *Diabetes.* https://www.diabetes.co.uk/diabetes-complications/poor-blood-circulation.html

Smoking and diabetes: What you should know. (n.d.). WebMD. https://www.webmd.com/diabetes/smoking-and-diabetes

Spritzler, F. (2020). How many carbs should you eat if you have diabetes? *Healthline Media.* https://www.healthline.com/nutrition/diabetes-carbs-per-day#daily-intake

Srakocic, S. (2022). Blood sugar level charts for type 1 and type 2 diabetes. *Healthline Media.* https://www.healthline.com/health/diabetes/blood-sugar-level-chart#recommended-ranges

Sherrell, Z. (2022). How do diabetes rates vary by country? *Medical News Today.* https://www.medicalnewstoday.com/articles/diabetes-rates-by-country

Steroids and diabetes: What you need to know. (2022). *Diabetes Daily.* https://www.diabetesdaily.com/learn-about-diabetes/treatment/other-drugs/steroids-and-diabetes-what-you-need-to-know/

Tello, C. (2019). 7 benefits of insulin & 2 negative effects. *SelfHacked.* https://selfhacked.com/blog/insulin-101/

Todd, J., Rudaizky, D., Clarke, P., & Sharpe, L. (2021). Cognitive biases in type 2 diabetes and chronic pan. *The Journal of Pain, 23*(1), 112–122. https://doi.org/10.1016/j.jpain.2021.06.016

The Diabetes Site. (2018, April 17). Diabetes and circulation: How to get the blood flowing again. *The Diabetes Site News.* https://blog.thediabetessite.greatergood.com/diabetes-circulation/

The Elderly and diabetes: Everything you need to know. (2016). TheDiabetesCouncil.Com. https://www.thediabetescouncil.com/the-elderly-and-diabetes-everything-you-need-to-know/

The Healthline Editorial Team. (2014). *How is type 2 diabetes diagnosed? What you need to know.* Healthline Media. https://www.healthline.com/health/type-2-diabetes/diagnosis#symptoms

The importance of exercise when you have diabetes. (2018). Harvard Health. https://www.health.harvard.edu/staying-healthy/the-importance-of-exercise-when-you-have-diabetes

The sweet danger of sugar. (2017). Harvard Health. https://www.health.harvard.edu/heart-health/the-sweet-danger-of-sugar

The unselfish art of prioritizing yourself. (2017). Psychology Today. https://www.psychologytoday.com/us/blog/compassion-matters/201708/the-unselfish-art-prioritizing-yourself

Tips for managing diabetes in the childcare setting. (n.d.). ADA. https://diabetes.org/tools-support/know-your-rights/safe-at-school-state-laws/special-considerations/tips-child-care-setting

Turbert, D. (2021). Diabetic eye disease. *American Academy of Ophthalmology.* https://www.aao.org/eye-health/diseases/diabetic-eye-disease

Type 2 diabetes. (n.d.). Diabetes UK. https://www.diabetes.org.uk/diabetes-the-basics/types-of-diabetes/type-2

Type 2 diabetes—Diagnosis and treatment. (2023). Mayo Clinic. https://www.mayoclinic.org/diseases-conditions/type-2-diabetes/diagnosis-treatment/drc-20351199

Understanding diagnosis and treatment of diabetes. (n.d.). WebMD. https://www.webmd.com/diabetes/news/20210629/best-blood-sugar-meds-for-type-2-diabetes

Vieira, G. (2018). How diabetes raises your risk for all major cancers. *Healthline Media.* https://www.healthline.com/health-news/diabetes-raises-risk-for-major-cancers

Watts, M. (2019). Diabetes and counting calories. *Diabetes.* https://www.diabetes.co.uk/features/diabetes-counting-calories.html

Weekly exercise targets. (n.d.). ADA. https://diabetes.org/healthy-living/fitness/weekly-exercise-targets

Weisenberger, J. (2023). *Lifestyle or Drugs to Control Diabetes? Which is Better?* https://jillweisenberger.com/lifestyle-changes-versus-drugs-diabetes-management/

What are some of the risk factors for type 2 diabetes? (2014). Healthline. https://www.healthline.com/health/type-2-diabetes-age-of-onset#risk-factors-for-adults

What are the most difficult challenges for diabetics? (n.d.). Quora. from https://www.quora.com/What-are-the-problems-faced-by-diabetes-patients

What can happen if my blood sugar is out of control? (n.d.). WebMD. https://www.webmd.com/diabetes/uncontrolled-blood-sugar-risks

What does a diabetic ulcer look like? (2019). https://www.medicalnewstoday.com/articles/320739

What high blood sugar does to your body. (n.d.). WebMD. https://www.webmd.com/diabetes/how-sugar-affects-diabetes

What is insulin resistance? A Mayo Clinic expert explains. (2022). [Video]. In *Mayo Clinic.* https://www.mayoclinic.org/diseases-conditions/obesity/multimedia/vid-20536756

Why Technology is Integral to Diabetes Care Management. (n.d.). HealthLeaders Media. rom https://www.healthleadersmedia.com/technology/why-technology-integral-diabetes-care-management

Woolley, E. (2012). How insulin works and why you need it. *Verywell Health.* https://www.verywellhealth.com/how-insulin-works-in-the-body-1087716

Woolston, C. (2020). Diabetes: Safety alerts and emergencies. *Consumer Health News | HealthDay.* https://consumer.healthday.com/encyclopedia/diabetes-13/diabetes-management-news-180/diabetes-safety-alerts-and-emergencies-644104.html

Wright, S. A. (2017). Everything you need to know about glucose. *Healthline Media.* https://www.healthline.com/health/glucose#What-is-glucose?

Yetman, D. (2021, June 23). What to know about diabetes and metabolism. *Healthline Media.* https://www.healthline.com/health/diabetes/diabetes-and-metabolism#metabolism-and-diabetes

BUILDING A COMMUNITY

"The best way to keep your blood pressure down is to know what makes it go up."

— MEISTER JOHANSEN

I'd like to ask you to take a moment to think about how you felt when you first received your diagnosis.

What emotions were running through you? Were you scared? Anxious? Overwhelmed? Did you ask yourself where you went wrong or if this was all your fault?

These are all common reactions to receiving a diagnosis of high blood pressure, and I've witnessed countless patients experience them. Suddenly being faced with a lifetime of monitoring and medication is overwhelming, and it can make you feel very isolated – even though you know that many other people are living with the condition.

This is why I'm committed to supporting as many people as possible – and to help me do that, I'd like to ask you to get involved.

The good news is, doing so will barely make a dent in your schedule, and you don't even have to leave your chair. All I'd like you to do is leave a review.

By leaving a review of this book on Amazon, you'll help other people living with high blood pressure feel less alone and point them in the direction of the support and guidance they're looking for.

Simply by telling new readers how this book has helped you and what they'll find inside, you'll help me to provide support for more people.

Thank you so much for your help. We can't reverse that feeling someone gets when they first receive their diagnosis, but we can help them to take control going forward. Together, we can build a community.

Scan the QR code below

UNDERSTANDING HIGH BLOOD PRESSURE

SIMPLE STEPS TO AVOID COMPLICATIONS, REDUCE MEDICAL EXPENSES, DECREASE STRESS, AND LIVE A HEALTHY & PROACTIVE LIFE

INTRODUCTION

"The doctor of the future will give no medication, but will interest his patients in the care of the human frame, diet and in the cause of prevention of disease"

— THOMAS EDISON

If you or a family member have been diagnosed with high blood pressure, you have a family history, or are just interested in learning more—you're in the right place!

High blood pressure or hypertension is a disease that can gradually progress. It can put you at risk for a stroke, kidney disease, or a heart attack. So, what can you do to prevent these from happening? You'll find various lists of tips and advice online. However, it's not as easy as it seems with the mountain of information you need to go through, and not knowing what information is reliable and credible.

As a person experiencing high blood pressure, you may be skeptical about your condition and the steps to control your blood pressure. As pharmacists, we find various patients battling hypertension, from physically strained workers to mentally stressed office employees. You may also know a relative who must take maintenance medications for their blood pressure. All around us people are trying to manage their blood pressure.

Even famous people like Larry King and Bill Clinton had to spend millions on expensive surgeries and procedures because of high blood pressure and heart complications. Bill Clinton had to lose weight and change his diet to legumes, beans, vegetables, and fruit. CNN interviewer Larry King had a heart attack, causing him to undergo bypass surgery. Blood pressure control is crucial to preventing these complications and procedures.

When you have hypertension, it means the pressure against your blood vessel walls is consistently too high. A blood pressure reading has two numbers: systolic and diastolic pressure. Systolic is the top number which measures blood pressure when the heart is contracting to move blood and diastolic is the bottom number which measures blood pressure when the heart is relaxed and filling with blood. These readings are categorized into ranges indicating whether you have a normal, mild, moderate, or hypertensive crisis, which we will further discuss within the chapters.

Since this disease has no obvious symptoms, many people don't know they have it until the condition has worsened. It is often known as a silent killer. Every individual will experience different symptoms, and most of the time, there are none. High blood pressure can be related to various causes. Nobody is safe from this genetic and lifestyle disease. Nevertheless, proper management and awareness can prevent serious consequences.

You may feel that life dealing with high blood pressure limits you from enjoying your favorite activities. However, many people manage to balance a healthy lifestyle, physical activity, and time with loved ones. You will get results and adapt to your condition with the proper knowledge and consistent effort.

Some patients wait for warning signs before making any changes, which is a dangerous practice. The best way to deal with high blood pressure is early intervention. You may hesitate to get a check-up with your doctor and find out about your results. But the sooner you get the right treatment plan, the better you can prevent further complications from developing. The cost of medications, diet changes, and doctor appointments may seem to be a heavy burden. Nonetheless, the earlier you take that step toward treatment, the less time and money you'll have to waste in the long run.

Different types of treatment plans are available for people with hypertension. Clinical guidelines are followed according to the American College of Cardiology and American Heart's Association (ACC/AHA). The prevalence of high blood pressure in 2015–2018 among adults in the U.S. shows that 116 million people had hypertension. Most of them are recommended medication and still do not have their hypertension under control. This is a great opportunity for education and lifestyle changes.

There are so many risk factors for heart disease and hypertension that affect every household and occupation. Job strain and blood pressure are significantly associated. It is essential to balance your job's physical demands if you have high blood pressure. Having to juggle work, social life, family, and blood pressure may feel overwhelming. You may worry about the sacrifices you have to make and feel impatient about the results.

Hypertension treatment will require you to change your lifestyle, but this does not imply your quality of life will be less. It requires you to make simple changes that give your health a chance, providing you with better opportunities to live fully into your later years. It will be worth all the sacrifices and patience in preventing life-threatening complications. Hypertension is one of the major causes of premature deaths worldwide. Reducing your blood pressure will also prevent other lifestyle diseases since it affects many organs including the heart, brain, and kidneys.

According to the World Health Organization (WHO), 46% of adults worldwide are undiagnosed. Hence, one of the global targets for non-communicable diseases is to reduce their prevalence by 33% between 2010 and 2030. A non-communicable disease is a disease that does not spread from person to person, it is the result of behavior, lifestyle, or genetic factors—not an acute illness.

Some patients with undiagnosed hypertension only learn about their condition after a heart attack resulting from severe hypertension. The risk of heart, brain, and kidney disease will demand more medications, leading to side effects and complications. Fortunately, numerous medications can help you control your hypertension. Although it may take time to find the correct dosage, coordinating with your healthcare professional will make the treatment successful. Moreover, several low-cost yet effective medications have been developed, and health insurance coverage can help you with expenses.

One check-up I witnessed at a clinic was from a patient that seemed physically active and only experienced occasional headaches, dizziness, and fatigue. He seemed like a healthy male in his 50s. He said he went on lengthy bike rides and crash diets to prevent weight gain. However, in between these routines, he would eat fatty foods and drink alcohol. He was surprised to find out that he was experiencing cardiomegaly or heart enlargement. This condition develops when the heart compensates for severe ongoing hypertension.

Another patient had their blood pressure under control after following their prescriptions and lifestyle changes. However, they stopped their medications when they felt their blood pressure was controlled. Some people assume that lifestyle changes are enough to treat all types of hypertension, but you must follow the instructions of your doctor if they advise you to take maintenance medications. Symptoms may return, and your condition may worsen if you stop treatment or return to unhealthy habits.

As previously mentioned, Larry King, a long-time smoker, quit on the day of his heart attack. He has since controlled his risk factors and built The Larry King Cardiac Foundation. David Letterman from *The Late Show*, whose father died of a heart attack, underwent quintuple bypass surgery. He had no complications after surgery and returned to hosting only after six weeks of recovery. These people went through complex procedures and improved their lifestyles. They have since been living their life fully. Many of them actively promote awareness and have supported foundations for cardiovascular diseases.

So how will you effectively monitor and manage your blood pressure? It may be challenging to know when you need to see your doctor. You may need help understanding how to measure your blood pressure initially, but you can get the hang of it quickly with the proper practice and information.

Furthermore, automated electronic monitors are available at pharmacies or online. These devices are much easier to use at home to keep track of your numbers.

For every condition, different types of medicines and lifestyle changes can be made. Whatever the cause of your hypertension and the dominant risks in your life, you will find the information you need in this book. It will provide step-by-step guidelines, descriptions, and answers to your questions. We will also debunk some misconceptions about hypertension.

This book will walk you through easily and successfully managing your condition. Learn about your symptoms, medications, lifestyle changes, and other ways to regulate your blood pressure. You will get optimal information and relatable stories from a healthcare provider's perspective translated into simple-to-understand words. Let's get started on your journey to understanding your body and all you need to know about managing high blood pressure.

1

UNDER PRESSURE

Did you know that high blood pressure is a common health concern, even among younger adults? Nearly 1 in 4 adults aged 20 to 44 have high blood pressure, which is a major risk factor for heart attack, stroke, and other serious health problems. Despite the prevalence of high blood pressure in this age group, it is often overlooked and undertreated. Understanding the importance of blood pressure and taking steps to monitor and control it early on can help prevent the development of serious health problems later in life.

OVERVIEW OF BLOOD PRESSURE

We know high blood pressure causes health issues, but what exactly does blood pressure measure? Blood pressure measures the force that moves blood against the walls of your arteries as the heart pumps blood. It is described as having two numbers: systolic and diastolic pressure. When your heart beats, it pumps blood into the circulatory system. Oxygen and nutrients are delivered throughout your body to nourish tissues and organs.

The blood exerts pressure on the arteries by forcing out blood when the heart contracts with every heartbeat. It beats 60 to 100 times a minute, 24 hours a day. The number of times your heart beats in one minute is called a heart rate. Blood pressure differs from heart rate because it measures how powerfully your blood travels through your blood vessels. They are both associated with the heart, but they measure different things. An increased heart rate doesn't mean your blood pressure is also increased.

Blood pressure changes as blood flows through the body. The circulatory system is like a form of plumbing. You could consider the arteries as pipes that follow the basic law of physics. The blood pressure is highest at the start and lowest at the end along smaller branches of arteries. The arteries can also be compared to the physical properties of a garden hose. If you squeeze a hose, the pressure on the walls where you constrict it increases.

The heart creates the maximum pressure for the blood to flow, but the properties of the arteries, such as their elasticity are also important. Hence, the condition of the arteries can affect blood pressure and flow. Moreover, if the arteries narrow, they can block the blood supply to the circulatory system.

If you want to monitor your blood pressure, you should be able to tell the normal blood pressure ranges. National guidelines provide parameters for normal and abnormal blood pressure levels. Blood pressure units are measured in millimeters of mercury or mm Hg. The National Institutes of Health and the American Heart Association (AHA) guidelines set the normal blood pressure below 120 mm Hg systolic and 80 mm Hg diastolic. Just remember, normal blood pressure is 120/80!

However, these guidelines have changed over the years. The older guidelines from 2003 were updated in 2017 and are currently being used. Since AHA followed the 2017 guidelines, it has allowed earlier intervention for people with high blood pressure.

Before the update, a prehypertension category existed between 120–139/80–89 mm Hg. Now, it is referred to as elevated blood pressure between 120–129/<80 mm Hg. People at risk of hypertension and in the earlier stages of hypertension are recommended lifestyle modifications. Moreover, people with 130–139 mm Hg/80–89 mm Hg qualify as stage 1 hypertension.

The numbers seem confusing at first, but with practice and guidance from your healthcare provider, you can get the hang of it. Blood pressure fluctuates based on different factors. Your blood pressure increases when you jog or ride a roller coaster. Yet, your blood pressure is lower when lying down or spending a day at the spa. Even age, medications, and changes in position affect your blood pressure. That's why there are certain guidelines followed when reading your blood pressure.

You may wonder why you need to know your blood pressure. When you get a check-up or go to a hospital, a healthcare provider will most likely ask for a reading. Blood pressure is the most commonly measured clinical parameter because it is a major determinant for diagnosis and treatment. Checking your blood pressure at every doctor visit allows for early detection and intervention to prevent further complications. This is especially important in those patients without symptoms of high blood pressure.

PHYSIOLOGY OF BLOOD PRESSURE REGULATION

Blood pressure regulation is a complex process that is operated by several mechanisms all at once. It gives insight into the working of the heart and vessels. If your body fails to regulate its blood pressure, it becomes too high or too low. This can lead to a wide range of diseases. This regulation mechanism is very important to maintaining healthy blood pressure to provide all organs with adequate blood supply and eliminate necessary waste.

Blood that gets delivered to the body picks up waste products and toxins. It regulates temperature and carries defending cells to tissue damage. Your heart, kidneys, and brain can become damaged if you have high blood pressure and your blood circulation does not function properly. High blood pressure is a major risk for complications and even fatal diseases.

Short-term adaptation and long-term maintenance of blood pressure are needed to keep it within a normal range. When your blood pressure needs rapid adjustments, it is regulated by a baroreceptor reflex. This reflex is a short-term regulation mechanism that influences the nervous (nerves) and endocrine (hormones) systems.

Higher blood pressure increases the activity of these baroreceptors. This increase reduces heart rate and the widening of blood vessels and arteries in order to lower blood pressure. However, when blood pressure decreases, receptor activity becomes lower. This reduction leads to an increased heart rate and vasoconstriction or narrowing of passages in order to raise blood pressure. These reactions adjust the blood pressure accordingly to keep it in the normal range.

The blood pressure regulation system keeps your blood pressure in a healthy range. Your heart, nervous system, hormones, and kidneys interact through the blood pressure regulation system. Your heart and kidneys work together and can affect each other's conditions. Therefore, if you have kidney disease, it can lead to heart disease and vice versa. In fact, they share many risk factors, such as diabetes and high blood pressure.

The heart pumps blood through your blood vessels, and the force of blood flow against the vessel walls is your blood pressure. The kidneys cleanse your blood and remove excess salt and water. This role makes it an important factor in regulating your blood pressure. It also helps control your blood volume and the diameter of blood vessels.

The kidney's other roles affecting blood pressure are regulating electrolytes and producing hormones. Without the kidneys, your blood would have too much waste and water. Without the heart, your kidneys won't have enough blood that delivers oxygen for them to function.

The impact of high blood pressure on the kidney is by constant stretching of small blood vessels in the kidney's tubules. The repeated stress on the vessel walls can cause scarring, leading to kidney problems. People with kidney disease fail to use the renin-angiotensin-aldosterone system (RAAS) system for blood regulation.

RAAS is a hormone system that can help regulate blood pressure and volume. Compared to the baroreceptor reflex, RAAS is slower but a long-term means of regulating blood pressure. The RAAS system relies on several hormones to increase blood volume and peripheral resistance. This resistance is used to create blood pressure and blood flow. When blood vessels constrict (vasoconstriction), it increases peripheral resistance—when blood vessels dilate (vasodilation), peripheral resistance decreases, and so does blood pressure.

When your blood pressure drops, the kidney secretes an enzyme called renin into the bloodstream. It is released when there is more salt in the blood, less blood flow in the kidney, or through the sympathetic nervous system. Renin is responsible for producing the angiotensin II hormone.

Angiotensin II causes vasoconstriction. Hence, the increase in angiotensin II can cause high blood pressure. Angiotensin II goes through different conversions, which starts off as angiotensinogen. Renin converts angiotensinogen to angiotensin I, eventually converted by the angiotensinogen-converting enzyme (ACE) into angiotensin II.

The names and terms may sound confusing, but you don't have to memorize them. Being familiar with and understanding how your body works can help you understand your condition and the medications you may use for treatment.

These processes create different responses that alter blood pressure. ACE, primarily from the lungs, also gets rid of bradykinin. Bradykinin is a vasodilator, which means it can widen the passage of blood. If it gets reduced, this leads to vasoconstriction or narrowing of passages.

Angiotensin II hormone will boost the release of the aldosterone hormone. Aldosterone will make the kidneys retain more salt and water, which results in more plasma volume and arterial pressure. Another way angiotensin II can increase plasma volume is through thirst and the antidiuretic hormone (ADH).

Aldosterone increases sodium while decreasing potassium and hydrogen through secretion in the kidneys. Since it can increase blood pressure through this process, several antihypertensive medications act through aldosterone.

This sequence of reactions is called the RAAS system. It efficiently and quickly increases blood pressure to maintain proper blood flow to vital organs. Since the RAAS system can increase blood volume and pressure, it can cause complications in certain individuals if it becomes overactive.

The cardiac cycle empties blood into the arterioles at an even rate, but the blood pressure undergoes natural variations from one heartbeat to another. Blood pressure changes in response to stress, nutritional factors, drugs, diseases, or position. The body regulates blood pressure by changes in response to the cardiac output and stroke volume.

When you suddenly stand up after lying down, your blood pressure temporarily increases. This rise ensures enough blood and oxygen gets to your brain. Changing positions can certainly impact your blood pressure.

When lying down, your heart doesn't have to pump so hard to circulate blood throughout your body. Most of your body parts are at the same level as your heart, which explains why you have lower blood pressure. Although minor changes in blood pressure exist, there is no medical consensus on the difference between positions.

A noticeable change in blood pressure is from lying down to standing up. Standing up causes the blood to pool in your lower body. Hence your blood pressure temporarily drops. This drop adjusts your body by making your heart beat faster to pump more blood, increasing your blood pressure. Occasionally you may feel this sudden drop in blood pressure when going to a standing position; this is called orthostatic hypotension.

Your blood pressure increases during exercise to help deliver more oxygen and nutrients to your muscles. This rise is usually temporary. Your blood pressure should gradually return to normal after exercise. During exercise, your systolic blood pressure increases more than diastolic. Your heart pumps harder and faster to circulate blood to the muscles. Since systolic represents the pressure when your heart beats and diastolic is when the heart rests, it may be concerning if the diastolic blood pressure significantly increases after exercising.

During exercise, your systolic blood pressure may rise between 160 and 220 mm Hg. Anywhere higher than 200 mm Hg should be discussed with a healthcare provider. A person with systolic blood pressure up to 250 mm Hg is considered to have exercise hypertension. Nevertheless, factors such as diet, drugs, and medical conditions may also affect how your heart responds to exercise.

Cardiac output, or the volume of blood pumped by the heart per minute, increases through an increased heart rate. This also happens when exercising. The blood vessels relax and widen during heavy exertion, offsetting the increased heart rate. This process regulates the amount of blood and oxygen going to your muscles. However, blood vessels narrow down when stressed, increasing blood pressure.

Your blood pressure fluctuates as a compensatory mechanism to help your body function properly. Blood pressure regulation has to maintain a high enough pressure that allows for blood flow to the organs and tissues but not too high that it causes harm. When your body goes through chronic hypertension, you can't pinpoint an exact cause. Rather, it is a consequence of the interaction of multiple risk factors.

Healthy arteries are smooth, and blood passes through easily. However, fats, cholesterol, and calcium can build up in the inner walls. This buildup, called plaque, slows blood flow, or may even block it. Blockages like plaque can make blood vessels too narrow and hardened to function properly. Blood pressure increases to compensate for this problem. Pressure increases to help push blood through the vessels, delivering proper blood flow to organs. However, it can lead to serious health problems if your body constantly compensates for different issues that affect your blood pressure.

There are no obvious symptoms at first, but they can develop as plaque builds up in the arteries. Usual signs are chest discomfort, dizziness, or excessive sweating. Since there is less blood supply to the legs and arms, it may cause pain and difficulty walking. Moreover, blocked arteries can lead to hypertension, stroke, or death. These serious consequences show us why it is so important to monitor your blood pressure and maintain a healthy lifestyle.

AN OVERWORKED HEART: THE DEFINITION AND CAUSES OF HIGH BLOOD PRESSURE

Hypertension is a medical term for chronic high blood pressure. High blood pressure or hypertension is when the force of blood pushing through your vessels is consistently too high. Blood vessels or arteries create resistance to blood flow when they become narrow. This effect leads to higher blood pressure.

Nearly half of American adults could be diagnosed with hypertension. It gradually develops over several years without being noticed. However, even without symptoms, hypertension can cause serious damage if left untreated. Early detection can be done with regular blood pressure readings. It is important to understand your blood pressure readings. Your doctor may ask you to check your blood pressure over a span of a few weeks or daily—depending on your condition.

High blood pressure causes damage to your tissues and organs. It starts in your arteries and heart. Your hypertension causes harm by increasing the workload of the heart and blood vessels, making them less efficient. This effect gradually damages the inner walls of the arteries. If the damage is prolonged, your hypertension worsens, leading to other harmful diseases.

Your blood pressure reading consists of two numbers. The top number is the systolic pressure when your heart beats and pumps blood. The bottom number is the diastolic pressure when your heart rests between beats.

There are currently five categories that define blood pressure readings.

- **Healthy** – comes in a blood pressure reading of less than 120/80 mm Hg.
- **Elevated** – is between 120–129 mm Hg for the top number and less than 80 mm Hg for the bottom number. Lifestyle changes are recommended for this category.
- **Stage 1 hypertension** – has a systolic pressure between 130–139 mm Hg and a diastolic pressure between 80–89 mm Hg.
- **Stage 2 hypertension** – has a reading equal to or higher than 140/90 mm Hg.

- **Hypertensive crisis** – is when your reading is over 180/120 mm Hg. Blood pressure within these numbers means you need urgent medical attention.

There are also different types of hypertension, called primary and secondary hypertension. They both result from high blood pressure. The difference between the two is the causes related to each. Primary hypertension doesn't have a conclusive or known cause, while secondary hypertension does. Nevertheless, they both lead to serious consequences if untreated.

There are key differences between the two. Primary hypertension occurs more often than secondary hypertension. Various risk factors increase your chances of developing it over the years. Unlike primary hypertension, secondary hypertension is rare and sudden. Moreover, it is caused by underlying conditions. The treatment plan for both may be taken with a different approach by your healthcare provider. Regardless, a healthy lifestyle is vital for both.

Primary Hypertension

Primary hypertension is also known as idiopathic or essential hypertension. It is a type of hypertension with multiple factors and doesn't have one distinct cause. The majority of people with high blood pressure have this type of hypertension. It is considered primary hypertension if none of the underlying causes of secondary hypertension exists. Your doctor will review your medical history and medications to rule this out.

According to the World Health Organization, 90–95% of adults have primary hypertension. It gradually develops through the years due to various factors. Since primary hypertension is not due to another medical condition, many causes are considered to manage it.

Risk factors include:

- Age (common in ages 65 years and older)
- Family history or genes
- Race
- Diet (high-salt intake)
- Obesity or being overweight
- Sedentary lifestyle or being inactive
- Stress
- Alcohol consumption
- Cigarette use

Secondary Hypertension

Secondary hypertension develops from an underlying condition, disease, or medication side effect. When high blood pressure is caused by a direct or distinct condition, it is considered secondary hypertension. According to the National Institute of Health, this rare type of hypertension occurs only in 2–10% of people with chronic high blood pressure. It is also known as resistant hypertension.

Common causes that are associated with it are:

- Kidney disease (damage to the kidneys can trigger the production of renin)
- Thyroid disease
- Adrenal disease (it causes hormone imbalance)
- Obstructive sleep apnea

- Oral contraceptives or birth control pills
- Nonsteroidal anti-inflammatory drugs (NSAIDs such as aspirin or ibuprofen)
- Antidepressants
- Decongestants
- Stimulants

Both primary and secondary hypertension usually occurs without specific symptoms. However, there are some indications of secondary hypertension, including the following:

- You are resistant to blood pressure medications, or they stop being effective.
- You develop hypertension suddenly with abrupt symptoms.
- Low potassium and high calcium levels.
- High creatinine levels.
- If you are at low risk but your blood pressure is too high. Nevertheless, people that are at high risk may still develop high blood pressure through secondary hypertension.

Primary and secondary hypertension can both exist when there is a sudden worsening of blood pressure. If a secondary cause is considered, additional tests such as kidney and heart ultrasound, electrocardiogram, and cholesterol screening may be conducted by your doctor. Physical signs indicating secondary hypertension include weight changes, swelling, abnormal hair growth, and stretch marks around the abdomen.

Moreover, secondary hypertension treatment options focus on the underlying issues diagnosed, such as kidney problems. If it is caused by a medication, an alternative may be recommended. Secondary hypertension has a positive outlook with treatment, especially if detected early. It will only last as long as you have the secondary condition.

Most cases of hypertension typically have no symptoms, even if your blood pressure becomes dangerously high. This is why it is often called a silent killer. It may cause damage to the body without you realizing it until your condition is severe or a heart attack occurs. Moreover, you can have high blood pressure for years without symptoms. It quietly causes damage that threatens your life.

A few people who experience symptoms may have headaches, shortness of breath, or nosebleeds. Nevertheless, the symptoms that take place will vary. They aren't specific and occur when your high blood pressure is at a life-threatening stage. According to the American Heart Association, nosebleeds and headaches don't happen until someone is in a hypertensive crisis.

Since many people are unaware that they have uncontrolled blood pressure, it is important to get regular blood pressure checks from a healthcare provider. When you visit a hospital or your doctor, they will get your blood pressure reading first. This is to ensure that it is within a healthy range. It also helps catch any potential issues early on.

Annual physicals and preventive maintenance are important for monitoring blood pressure. It can help detect and address potential problems before they become more serious. Your healthcare provider can discuss your risks and other readings to help monitor your blood pressure.

Hypertension can cause various damages to the body. Complications with your organs and other body functions will interfere with your quality of life. The damage high blood pressure can inflict may lead to life-threatening complications. It often has a domino effect of consequences on your health. High blood pressure can lead to the following:

Damage to the heart and arteries

High blood pressure causes strain on the heart, leading to enlargement and other issues. It increases the workload on your circulatory system, failing to supply blood efficiently. Arteries should be flexible, strong, and elastic, while blood is supposed to flow smoothly through the arteries. It should efficiently supply nutrients and oxygen to your body.

- Heart attack – high blood pressure narrows and stiffens the arteries, which increases the risk of a heart attack.

- Heart failure – the strain on the heart can cause the heart muscle to weaken and fail.
- Coronary artery disease – when the blood supply to the heart is affected by decreased blood flow, it leads to chest pain (angina) or irregular heart rhythms (arrhythmias).
- Peripheral artery disease (PAD) – damaged arteries can lead to atherosclerosis. This condition limits blood flow to the legs, arms, stomach, and head, causing pain or fatigue.
- Damaged and narrowed arteries – damaged arteries can collect fats or plaque, making the artery walls narrow and hardened.
- Aneurysm – it is when a section of an artery wall becomes enlarged and forms a bulge. This bulge or aneurysm can rupture and cause internal bleeding.

Damage to the brain

The brain needs blood and oxygen supply to function properly. High blood pressure and heart problems can cause life-threatening brain damage.

- Stroke – if your hypertension worsens, blood vessels in the brain are damaged. The clogged blood vessels in the brain block blood flow, leading to stroke.
- Transient ischemic attack (TIA) – it is sometimes called a ministroke, which is also a warning sign for a full-blown stroke. TIA is a brief, temporary

interruption of blood supply to the brain due to hardened arteries or blood clots.
- Dementia – when the blood flow to the brain is limited, it leads to vascular dementia.
- Mild cognitive impairment – this is the transition between the normal part of aging and dementia, which affects understanding and memory.

Damage to the kidneys

Hypertension affects the crucial role of the kidney in filtering blood, which requires healthy blood vessels.

- Kidney scarring – is when tiny blood vessels linked to the kidney become scarred, leading to kidney failure. It is also known as glomerulosclerosis.
- Kidney failure – high blood pressure can damage the arteries in the kidneys. When blood isn't filtered properly, dangerous levels of fluid and waste accumulate in the blood.

Damage to the eyes

The eyes have tiny, delicate blood vessels. If these vessels are strained or damaged, the following may occur:

- Retinopathy – is caused by damaged blood vessels in the retina. The retina is the light-sensitive tissue at the back of your eyes. This can lead to bleeding, blurred vision, and total vision loss.

- Choroidopathy – is the fluid buildup under the retina, causing distorted vision. It can also cause scarring.
- Optic neuropathy – it is also known as nerve damage. The optic nerve can be damaged when blood flow is blocked, leading to bleeding and vision loss.

Sexual dysfunction

Hypertension can reduce blood flow to the body, including the genitals. Their function is impaired due to limited blood flow and oxygen.

- Erectile dysfunction – men may have difficulty maintaining or having an erection as they age. High blood pressure increases their risk of experiencing this.
- Lower libido – women may experience a decreased sex drive, vaginal dryness, and difficulty having an orgasm.

The prevalence of hypertension per age group

The prevalence of hypertension is a major public health challenge in the United States because of its consequences on people's quality of life. The number of adults with hypertension in 2015–2016 was 29%. This increases with age, as it is a risk factor for high blood pressure. There were 7.5% of adults between 18–39 who had hypertension. For ages 40–59, it hiked to 33.2%. Lastly, those aged 60 and over had a 63.1% prevalence of hypertension.

MEASURING AND DIAGNOSING

Measuring your blood pressure is an important routine that you should learn. Consistently monitoring it helps you control your blood pressure. You can ask a family member to help you keep track. We often find older people who repeatedly measure their blood pressure when they feel distressed. Most often, it is better to calm them down before taking that reading. The following information will guide you in measuring someone else's or your own blood pressure:

A blood pressure reading is taken with a cuff or a sphygmomanometer. This strap-like device is used by your doctor for a more accurate reading.

A blood pressure reading tests the force exerted on the arteries. It is measured in millimeters of mercury (mm Hg), including the below two readings:

- Systolic blood pressure is found first or at the top of the denomination. Systolic pressure is the force inside the artery walls as the heart beats.

- Diastolic blood pressure is the second or lower denomination in a blood pressure reading. Diastolic pressure is when the heart is at rest.

A blood pressure measurement can be used to diagnose hypertension in its early stages. High blood pressure usually doesn't have warning signs or symptoms, so regularly measuring your blood pressure helps you get treated early.

It is the primary test for screening hypertension in a patient. A blood pressure measurement is often required when you get a regular check-up at your doctor or the hospital. It is recommended that adults have their blood pressure tested every few years or yearly if they are at risk.

You may be familiar with these steps in measuring blood pressure if you've been to the hospital or for a health check-up:

- A nurse or healthcare provider will ask you to sit in a chair with your feet flat on the ground.
- Your arm should rest on a table at your heart's level.
- The blood pressure cuff is wrapped around your upper arm to fit just right, with the bottom edge of the cuff placed just above your elbow.
- Using a small hand pump or a button, the cuff wrapped around your arm will be inflated.

- If a manual blood pressure cuff is used, your healthcare provider will use a stethoscope to listen to your blood flow and pulse.
- While the cuff inflates, it will tighten around your arm. And as it deflates, the blood pressure falls.
- When the blood pressure falls, the sound of blood pulsing is first heard. This is recorded as systolic pressure.
- The blood pulsing sound disappears, and the cuff's air is released. Once the sound completely stops, it is recorded as diastolic pressure.
- An automated device will display a digital reading after inflating and deflating on its own.

Your blood pressure may be slightly affected by factors such as medications, caffeine, physical activity, emotional state, and the time of the day. Nevertheless, there are no preparations before taking your blood pressure. It is recommended to monitor your blood pressure frequently, particularly in the morning as you wake up.

After taking your blood pressure, you must record your results. This will contain your systolic and diastolic pressure. You can check the chart for the categories of hypertension to determine if your blood pressure is under control. Your doctor will provide a diagnosis and treatment plan based on your blood pressure readings. If you track your blood pressure at home, it is good practice to keep a notebook to log your readings and bring them to your visits with your physician or pharmacist.

A diagnosis of elevated blood pressure is determined with two or more blood pressure readings. They may recommend home monitoring with an automated blood pressure device. However, you will still be required to visit your doctor regularly. Monitoring your blood pressure will help update or optimize your treatment.

If you suspect you or a family member has high blood pressure, an appointment with a doctor should be scheduled. Testing your blood pressure only takes a few minutes. A blood pressure screening is a painless procedure. However, some other tests and procedures may be requested. Your doctor will check for causes of high blood pressure and assess the risk from the condition or the treatment. Procedures and tests included in the diagnosis are:

- Blood tests or complete blood count (CBC)

  - Electrolytes
  - Blood urea nitrogen (BUN)
  - Creatinine levels (to assess kidney issues)

- Lipid profile for cholesterol
- Glucose test for blood sugar
- Special tests for hormones (to assess adrenal or thyroid issues)
- Urine tests for electrolytes and hormones
- Eye examination with an ophthalmoscope (to assess ocular damage)
- Ultrasound of kidneys
- CT scan of the abdomen

For people with severe hypertension, damage to the heart or blood vessels should be determined with the following tests:

- Electrocardiogram (ECG) – detects the electrical activity of the heart. ECG evaluates the damage to the heart muscles.
- Echocardiogram – an ultrasound examination of the heart through the chest. An echocardiogram will detect abnormalities in your heart size, heart wall, heart valve, and blood clots. Moreover, it can measure the strength of the heart muscle. It is more comprehensive than ECG but also costly.

- Chest X-ray – a simple procedure that provides an estimated heart size.
- Doppler ultrasound – checks the blood flow through the arteries in your arms, legs, hands, and feet. It detects peripheral vascular disease caused by the narrowing of arteries.

Since hypertension usually doesn't have symptoms, your doctor will ask about your medical records, current medications, family history, vices, and other risk factors. In addition, a physical exam is conducted using a stethoscope. In addition, your doctor will listen to your heartbeat for any abnormalities. They may also check for your pulse to see if they are weak or absent.

Now that you have a solid understanding of blood pressure and hypertension, it's important to dive deeper into the risk factors contributing to developing high blood pressure.

2

WHAT PUTS YOU AT RISK FOR HIGH BLOOD PRESSURE?

Did you know that hypertension impacts over 30% of the global adult population, affecting more than one billion individuals? It serves as the primary risk factor for various cardiovascular conditions, including coronary heart disease and stroke, as well as chronic kidney disease, heart failure, arrhythmia, and dementia.

In this chapter, I will be walking you through the risk factors associated with hypertension. Read on to find out how you, or somebody you care about, could be harboring habits that are impacting their health.

RISK FACTORS FOR HIGH BLOOD PRESSURE

Understanding the risk factors for high blood pressure is essential for effective prevention and management of hypertension. Various factors contribute to an individual's risk of developing high blood pressure, including age, gender, genetics, and lifestyle choices. By gaining a deeper understanding of these risk factors, individuals can make informed decisions to minimize their risk and maintain optimal cardiovascular health.

1. Age: The risk of developing high blood pressure increases as we age. With time, blood vessels can lose their elasticity, which can contribute to increased resistance and higher blood pressure levels. According to the American Heart Association, nearly two-thirds of adults over 60 years old have high blood pressure. However, younger individuals are not immune to hypertension, and it is essential to monitor blood pressure levels and adopt healthy lifestyle habits early in life.

2. Gender: There are differences in the prevalence of high blood pressure between men and women. Men are generally more likely to develop hypertension at a younger age, while women's risk increases significantly after menopause. Estrogen is believed to play a protective role against hypertension in premenopausal women, but this protection diminishes with age. Regardless of gender, it is crucial to be proactive about blood pressure management and adopt lifestyle changes that promote heart health.

3. Genetics: Family history and genetics can significantly influence an individual's risk of developing high blood pressure. If one or both of your parents have hypertension, your risk of developing the condition is higher. Although you cannot change your genetic predisposition, understanding your family history can help you make more informed decisions about your lifestyle and healthcare to mitigate your risk.

4. Lifestyle factors: A wide range of lifestyle factors can contribute to high blood pressure, including:

> a. **Poor diet**: Consuming a diet high in salt, saturated fats, and processed foods can increase blood pressure levels. Adopting a heart-healthy diet, such as the DASH (Dietary Approaches to Stop Hypertension) diet, which emphasizes whole grains, fruits, vegetables, lean proteins, and low-fat dairy products, can help lower blood pressure, and maintain optimal cardiovascular health.
> b. **Physical inactivity**: Leading a sedentary lifestyle can contribute to weight gain, decreased cardiovascular fitness, and increased blood pressure levels. Engaging in regular physical activity, such as walking, swimming, or cycling, can help lower blood pressure, improve heart health, and promote overall well-being.
> c. **Excessive alcohol consumption:** Drinking alcohol in moderation (one drink per day for women and up to two drinks per day for men) may have some cardiovascular benefits. However, excessive alcohol consumption can lead to weight gain, liver damage, and increased blood pressure levels. Limiting alcohol

intake can help prevent hypertension and promote better overall health.

d. **Stress**: Chronic stress can elevate blood pressure levels by causing the release of stress hormones, which can constrict blood vessels and increase heart rate. Developing effective stress management techniques, such as deep breathing exercises, meditation, and yoga, and engaging in hobbies or activities that promote relaxation and enjoyment, can help manage blood pressure and promote overall well-being.

Apart from these, obesity, a sedentary lifestyle, tobacco use, smoking, and certain medical conditions are all significant risk factors as well. Let's delve deeper into these risk factors and their impact on hypertension:

1. Obesity: Excess body weight, particularly around the abdomen, increases the risk of high blood pressure. Obesity can cause the heart to work harder to pump blood, leading to increased pressure on the arterial walls. Additionally, obesity is often associated with other health issues such as sleep apnea, diabetes, and high cholesterol, which can further contribute to hypertension. Implementing a weight loss plan through healthy dietary changes and regular physical activity can help lower blood pressure and reduce the risk of complications.

2. Sedentary lifestyle: A lack of physical activity can lead to weight gain and decreased cardiovascular fitness, both of which contribute to high blood pressure. Physical inactivity may also result in the weakening of the heart muscle, which can lead to a less efficient pumping action and elevated blood pressure. Incorporating regular exercise into your daily routine can improve heart health, lower blood pressure, and promote overall well-being.

3. Tobacco use: Tobacco use, including smoking and smokeless tobacco products, can cause a temporary increase in blood pressure and damage the cardiovascular system over time. The chemicals found in tobacco can narrow blood vessels and increase arterial stiffness, leading to elevated blood pressure levels. Quitting tobacco use and avoiding exposure to secondhand smoke can significantly reduce the risk of hypertension and its associated complications.

4. Smoking: Similar to tobacco use, smoking can cause both short-term and long-term increases in blood pressure. The nicotine in cigarettes can constrict blood vessels, increase heart rate, and elevate blood pressure temporarily. Over time, smoking can damage blood vessels and contribute to the development of atherosclerosis, further increasing the risk of hypertension. Quitting smoking is one of the most effective ways to lower blood pressure and improve cardiovascular health.

5. Sleep apnea: Sleep apnea is a medical condition characterized by repeated interruptions in breathing during sleep, leading to decreased oxygen levels in the blood. This can cause the release of stress hormones, increased heart rate, and elevated blood pressure. Treating sleep apnea with continuous positive airway pressure (CPAP) therapy or other appropriate interventions can help lower blood pressure and reduce the risk of hypertension-related complications.

6. Kidney disease: The kidneys play a crucial role in regulating blood pressure by filtering blood and removing excess salt and water. When the kidneys are damaged or not functioning properly, they may be unable to remove excess salt and water effectively, leading to increased blood volume and elevated blood pressure. Proper management of kidney disease, including medication and lifestyle changes, can help control blood pressure and prevent further kidney damage.

7. Diabetes: Individuals with diabetes are at a higher risk of developing high blood pressure due to the effects of high blood sugar levels on blood vessels and the kidneys. Over time, elevated blood sugar can damage blood vessels, making them less flexible and more prone to narrowing, leading to increased blood pressure. Additionally, diabetes can impact kidney function, further contributing to hypertension. Managing diabetes through medication, diet, and exercise is essential for maintaining healthy blood pressure levels and preventing complications.

Understanding and addressing these risk factors can significantly reduce an individual's risk of developing high blood pressure and its associated complications. By adopting a healthy lifestyle, staying physically active, maintaining a balanced diet, managing stress, and limiting alcohol intake, individuals can effectively manage their blood pressure levels and improve their overall cardiovascular health.

In essence, taking control of one's lifestyle and understanding the various risk factors for high blood pressure is critical for effective prevention and management of hypertension. By making informed decisions about diet, exercise, stress management, and other lifestyle factors, individuals can reduce their risk of developing high blood pressure and maintain optimal cardiovascular health. Regular check-ups with a healthcare provider can also help identify any potential issues early on and ensure that appropriate interventions are implemented to maintain healthy blood pressure.

SUPPORTING FACTORS

Environmental factors can also contribute to the development of high blood pressure, including stress, certain medications, and pregnancy. Understanding the impact of these factors on blood pressure levels is essential for effective management and prevention of hypertension.

1. Stress: Chronic stress can have a significant impact on blood pressure by causing the release of stress hormones, which can constrict blood vessels and increase heart rate. While short-term stress may lead to temporary spikes in blood pressure, long-term stress can contribute to sustained hypertension. It is important to identify and manage stressors in one's life to maintain healthy blood pressure levels.

2. Medication: Certain medications can contribute to high blood pressure, either as a direct side effect or through interactions with other medications or substances. Common medications that may affect blood pressure include decongestants, nonsteroidal anti-inflammatory drugs (NSAIDs), oral contraceptives, and certain antidepressants. It is crucial to discuss potential side effects and interactions with your healthcare provider before starting any new medication and to monitor your blood pressure closely while taking medications that may impact it. If you suspect that a medication may be contributing to your high blood pressure, speak with your healthcare provider about possible alternatives or adjustments to your treatment plan.

3. Pregnancy: High blood pressure can develop during pregnancy, either as a pre-existing condition (chronic hypertension) or as a pregnancy-related complication (gestational hypertension or preeclampsia). Pregnant women with high blood pressure are at an increased risk of complications for both themselves and their babies, including preterm birth, low birth weight, and placental abruption. It is essential for women with high blood pressure to receive appropriate prenatal care and work closely with their healthcare providers to monitor and manage their blood pressure throughout pregnancy. In some cases, medication may be prescribed to help control blood pressure levels, while in others, lifestyle changes, such as dietary modifications and exercise may be recommended.

4. Environmental factors: Exposure to certain environmental factors, such as air pollution and noise pollution, has been linked to increased blood pressure levels. Long-term exposure to air pollution, particularly particulate matter, can cause inflammation and oxidative stress, leading to blood vessel damage and elevated blood pressure. Similarly, chronic exposure to high noise levels, especially during nighttime, can contribute to stress and disrupt sleep patterns, both of which can impact blood pressure. To minimize the effects of these environmental factors on blood pressure, consider using air purifiers, noise-canceling headphones, or other strategies to reduce exposure to air and noise pollution.

Remember, understanding blood pressure, its risk factors, and the role of environmental factors is crucial in managing hypertension effectively. By adopting a healthy lifestyle, addressing potential risk factors, and staying vigilant about the impact of stress, medication, and pregnancy on blood pressure levels, individuals can significantly reduce their risk of developing high blood pressure and its associated complications.

In the next chapter, we will explore various medications and strategies to avoid potential interactions with other drugs or supplements. Staying informed and working closely with your healthcare provider will empower you to find the best treatment plan to manage your high blood pressure and enhance your overall well-being.

3

MEDICATIONS FOR MANAGING HIGH BLOOD PRESSURE

As we embark on this new chapter of our journey together, I'd like to take a moment to discuss the diverse range of medications available for managing high blood pressure and offer some guidance on steering clear of harmful drug interactions. You might be surprised to learn that the simultaneous use of multiple medications, a phenomenon referred to as polypharmacy, can significantly increase the likelihood of experiencing adverse reactions.

It's a curious fact that the more medications we introduce into our systems, the greater the chances of encountering harmful drug interactions. Studies have demonstrated that patients who take between five and nine medications face a 50% probability of experiencing an adverse drug interaction. Even more staggering is that this risk skyrockets to a complete 100% when an individual takes twenty or more medications concurrently.

Moreover, as stated by Health Research Funding, almost 30% of all hospital admissions can be attributed to polypharmacy, making it the fifth leading cause of death in the United States. That's correct—the excessive consumption of medications can pose a severe and potentially fatal risk to our well-being.

As we delve deeper into this chapter, I aim to provide original, insightful information on managing high blood pressure through various medications. Remember the importance of vigilance and caution when avoiding the dangerous territory of harmful drug interactions.

Medications undoubtedly play a vital role in the quest to manage high blood pressure, a widespread and potentially severe health concern. High blood pressure, if left unaddressed, can lead to various complications, such as heart disease, stroke, and kidney failure. Identifying the most effective medications to control this condition is important.

Various medications are available for treating high blood pressure, each working through distinct mechanisms to maintain healthy blood pressure levels. Some of these medications function by reducing fluid volume within the body, thereby lessening the pressure exerted on blood vessels. Others operate by relaxing the blood vessels, enabling smoother blood flow, and reducing pressure. Yet another category of high blood pressure medications targets specific hormones that contribute to elevated blood pressure, effectively blocking their impact.

Collaborating closely with a healthcare provider is essential to ascertain the most suitable medication or combination of medications tailored to an individual's unique needs. Medical professionals possess the necessary expertise to assess each patient's medical history, current health condition, and other factors that may influence the choice of medication. It is crucial to remember that managing high blood pressure is not a one-size-fits-all approach, and a healthcare provider can help determine the most effective treatment plan for each person.

Once the appropriate medication or combination of medications has been prescribed, it is important to follow the healthcare provider's instructions closely. This includes taking the medications as prescribed, adhering to the recommended dosages, and maintaining a consistent schedule. Deviating from the prescribed regimen may reduce effectiveness and potentially exacerbate the underlying condition.

In addition to following the prescribed treatment plan, monitoring any potential side effects or interactions with other medications is crucial. As discussed earlier, the risk of harmful drug interactions increases with the number of medications being taken concurrently. Consequently, it is vital to maintain open communication with your healthcare provider about all medications you are currently taking, including over-the-counter drugs, supplements, and herbal remedies. This will enable the healthcare provider to evaluate the potential for interactions and adjust the medication regimen if necessary.

Furthermore, being proactive in identifying and reporting any side effects that may arise while taking high blood pressure medications is essential. Some side effects might be temporary and resolved independently, while others could be more serious and require medical intervention. By closely monitoring your body's response to the medications, you can help your healthcare provider make informed decisions about your treatment plan and ensure your safety and well-being.

HOW DO BLOOD PRESSURE MEDICINES WORK?

Blood pressure medicines, known as antihypertensives, are designed to regulate and lower high blood pressure. These medications function through various mechanisms, targeting different aspects of the cardiovascular system to maintain healthy blood pressure. Here are some of the primary ways in which these medicines work:

1. **Diuretics**: These medications, sometimes called "water pills," aid the kidneys in removing excess sodium and water from the body. This fluid volume reduction decreases blood vessel pressure, ultimately lowering blood pressure.

2. **Beta-blockers**: By blocking the effects of the hormone epinephrine, also known as adrenaline, beta-blockers help slow down the heart rate and reduce the force with which the heart pumps blood. This results in decreased blood pressure.
3. **Calcium channel blockers**: These medications inhibit the movement of calcium into the muscle cells of the heart and blood vessels. This action relaxes the blood vessels and reduces the force of the heart's contractions, leading to a decline in blood pressure.
4. **ACE inhibitors**: Angiotensin-converting enzyme (ACE) inhibitors prevent the production of angiotensin II, a hormone that causes blood vessels to constrict. ACE inhibitors promote the relaxation of blood vessels by inhibiting this hormone and effectively lowering blood pressure. Remember the RAAS system from earlier?
5. **Angiotensin II receptor blockers (ARBs)**: Similar to ACE inhibitors, ARBs block the action of angiotensin II but do so by preventing it from binding to its receptors. This interference results in relaxed blood vessels and decreased blood pressure.
6. **Alpha-blockers**: Alpha-blockers relax blood vessels to reduce resistance in blood flow.
7. **Alpha-beta blockers**: Combined alpha-beta blockers are often used in hypertensive crises and are given through an IV drip. They also have an oral form used

in patients who are at risk for heart failure or in pregnancy.
8. **Central-acting agents**: Central agonists reduce tension in the blood vessels.
9. **Vasodilators**: Blood vessel dilators relax the muscle in the blood vessel wall, allowing the vessels to widen and improve blood flow.
10. **Aldosterone receptor antagonists**: ARAs inhibit the hormone aldosterone and promote the excretion of sodium and water and the retention of potassium, helping to reduce blood volume and lowering blood pressure.
11. **Direct renin inhibitors**: Directly inhibiting renin, an enzyme that triggers a sequence of reactions leading to blood vessel constriction and sodium retention, helps relax blood vessels, and reduces fluid retention.

WHAT ARE THE BENEFITS AND RISKS OF BLOOD PRESSURE MEDICINES?

In this section, I will walk you through the benefits of blood pressure medications. Read on to find out more.

Benefits:

1. High blood pressure, if left untreated, can lead to several severe health issues, such as heart attack,

stroke, kidney disease, and vision loss. Blood pressure medicines help minimize the risk of these complications by effectively managing the condition.
2. Properly controlled blood pressure enables individuals to lead healthier and more active lives without the constant worry of potential complications arising from elevated blood pressure.
3. Blood pressure medicines not only lower blood pressure but also contribute to overall heart health by reducing the strain on the heart and blood vessels.

Risks:

1. As with any medication, blood pressure medicines can cause side effects. These may range from mild and temporary to more severe and persistent.
2. In some cases, blood pressure medication may lower blood pressure too much, causing hypotension (abnormally low blood pressure). This may result in dizziness, fainting, or even shock.
3. Combining blood pressure medicines with other medications, supplements, or herbal remedies can sometimes lead to harmful interactions, which may reduce the efficacy of the treatment or cause adverse reactions.

WHAT ARE THE COMMON SIDE EFFECTS OF BLOOD PRESSURE MEDICINES?

The common side effects of blood pressure medicines vary depending on the specific medication and the individual's response to the treatment. Some common side effects include:

1. **Dizziness or lightheadedness:** This may occur when the blood pressure drops too quickly, causing a temporary reduction in blood flow to the brain.
2. **Fatigue:** Some blood pressure medications, particularly beta-blockers, may cause feelings of tiredness or fatigue.
3. **Dry cough:** ACE inhibitors are known to cause a persistent dry cough in some individuals. In these patients, an ARB is a good alternative.
4. **Swelling in the legs, ankles, or feet:** Calcium channel blockers may cause fluid retention, leading to swelling in the lower extremities.
5. **Erectile dysfunction:** Some blood pressure medicines, such as diuretics and beta-blockers, may contribute to erectile dysfunction in men.
6. **Gastrointestinal issues:** Nausea, diarrhea, or constipation may occur as side effects of some blood pressure medications.
7. **Headaches:** Some individuals may experience headaches as a side effect of blood pressure

medicines, particularly when starting a new medication or adjusting the dosage.
8. **Insomnia:** Certain blood pressure medications, such as beta-blockers, may cause difficulty falling or staying asleep.
9. **Skin rash:** In some cases, individuals may develop a skin rash or sensitivity to sunlight while taking blood pressure medicines.
10. **Weight gain**: Some blood pressure medications, particularly beta-blockers, may cause weight gain due to fluid retention or changes in metabolism.

It's essential to discuss any side effects you experience with your healthcare provider. In many cases, side effects can be managed or resolved by adjusting the medication dosage or switching to a different medication.

HOW DO YOU KNOW IF YOU NEED MEDICINE FOR HIGH BLOOD PRESSURE?

Determining whether you need medicine for high blood pressure involves several factors, including your blood pressure levels, overall health, and the presence of other risk factors or conditions.

1. Healthcare providers use specific guidelines to determine whether an individual requires medication for high blood pressure. Generally, if your blood pressure consistently measures 140/90 mm Hg or higher, your healthcare provider may consider prescribing medication.
2. If your blood pressure is mildly elevated, your healthcare provider may recommend lifestyle changes, such as a healthy diet, regular exercise, weight loss, stress management, and reducing alcohol and tobacco consumption. If these lifestyle modifications are insufficient in lowering blood pressure, medication may become necessary.
3. If you have other health conditions, such as diabetes, kidney disease, or heart disease, your healthcare provider may prescribe medication to manage your blood pressure more aggressively, even if it's only mildly elevated. This approach is aimed at reducing the risk of complications associated with high blood pressure.

4. Older individuals may require medication to manage their blood pressure, as the risk of complications increases with age.
5. If you have a family history of high blood pressure or related complications, your healthcare provider may recommend medication as a preventive measure.

It's essential to work closely with your healthcare provider to determine the most appropriate course of action for managing your high blood pressure. Regular blood pressure monitoring, medical checkups, and open communication with your healthcare provider will ensure that you receive the most effective treatment plan tailored to your individual needs.

CLASSES OF BLOOD PRESSURE MEDICATIONS

As we navigate through the world of blood pressure medications, it's essential to understand the various classes of these medicines. Each class has a distinct mechanism of action, which determines how they help control blood pressure. I will guide you through the different classes, discussing their mechanisms and possible side effects and providing examples for each. Let's begin!

1. Diuretics

Diuretics, sometimes known as "water pills," work by helping the kidneys expel excess water and sodium from the body. By reducing fluid volume, these medications decrease the pressure exerted on blood vessels, ultimately lowering blood pressure. There are several types of diuretics which include thiazides, potassium-sparing, loop, and combination. Each category works on a different area within the kidneys. You may be prescribed multiple diuretics from different categories. Many of these medications deplete potassium levels except for potassium-sparing diuretics. It is important to maintain potassium in your diet or supplements to prevent weakness, fatigue, and muscle cramps.

Possible side effects:

- Increased urination
- Dizziness or lightheadedness
- Electrolyte imbalances (such as low potassium levels)
- Dehydration
- Fatigue
- Muscle cramps

Examples:

Thiazide Diuretics

- Chlorthalidone

- Hydrochlorothiazide (Microzide)
- Indapamide
- Metolazone (Zaroxolyn)

Potassium-Sparing Diuretics

- Amiloride
- Spironolactone (Aldactone)
- Triamterene
- Eplerenone (Inspra)

Loop Diuretics

- Furosemide (Lasix)
- Bumetanide (Bumex)

Combination Diuretics

- Amiloride + Hydrochlorothiazide (Moduretic)
- Spironolactone + Hydrochlorothiazide (Aldactazide)
- Triamterene + Hydrochlorothiazide (Maxzide, Dyazide)

2. Beta-blockers

Beta-blockers function by blocking the effects of the hormone epinephrine (adrenaline), which helps slow down the heart rate and reduce the force with which the heart pumps blood. Consequently, this results in decreased blood pressure.

Possible side effects:

- Fatigue or lethargy
- Cold hands and feet
- Dizziness or lightheadedness
- Dry mouth, eyes, or skin
- Insomnia
- Weight gain
- Erectile dysfunction

Examples:

- Atenolol (Tenormin)
- Bisoprolol (Zebeta)
- Metoprolol tartrate (Lopressor)
- Metoprolol succinate (Toprol-XL)
- Propranolol (Inderal)
- Sotalol (Betapace)
- Nadolol (Corgard)
- Acebutolol (Sectral)

Combination Beta-Blocker and Thiazide Diuretic

- Bisoprolol + Hydrochlorothiazide (Ziac)

3. Calcium channel blockers

Calcium channel blockers inhibit the movement of calcium into the muscle cells of the heart and blood vessels. By doing so, these medications relax the blood vessels and reduce the force of the heart's contractions, leading to a decline in blood pressure.

Possible side effects:

- Swelling in the legs, ankles, or feet
- Constipation
- Headaches
- Dizziness or lightheadedness
- Flushing or redness in the face
- Rapid or irregular heartbeat (palpitations)

Examples:

- Amlodipine (Norvasc)
- Diltiazem (Cardizem)
- Felodipine (Plendil)
- Nifedipine (Procardia, Adalat)
- Verapamil (Calan, Verelan)
- Nicardipine (Cardene)

4. ACE inhibitors

Angiotensin-converting enzyme (ACE) inhibitors work by preventing the production of angiotensin II, a hormone that causes blood vessels to constrict. This inhibition results in the relaxation of blood vessels, effectively lowering blood pressure. It is important to note that pregnant women should not take ACE Inhibitors.

Possible side effects:

- Dry, persistent cough
- Dizziness or lightheadedness
- Headaches
- Fatigue
- Swelling in the face or throat (angioedema)
- Elevated potassium levels (hyperkalemia)

Examples:

- Benazepril (Lotensin)
- Captopril (Capoten)
- Enalapril (Vasotec)
- Lisinopril (Prinivil, Zestril)
- Ramipril (Altace)
- Fosinopril (Monopril)
- Quinapril (Accupril)

5. Angiotensin II receptor blockers (ARBs)

Angiotensin II receptor blockers (ARBs) block the action of angiotensin II by preventing it from binding to its receptors. This interference results in relaxed blood vessels and decreased blood pressure, much like ACE inhibitors. It is important to note that pregnant women should not take ARBs.

Possible side effects:

- Dizziness or lightheadedness
- Headaches
- Fatigue
- Elevated potassium levels (hyperkalemia)
- Swelling in the face or throat (angioedema)—although this is less common than with ACE inhibitors.

Examples:

- Losartan (Cozaar)
- Valsartan (Diovan)
- Irbesartan (Avapro)
- Candesartan (Atacand)
- Olmesartan (Benicar)
- Telmisartan (Micardis)

6. Alpha-blockers

Alpha-blockers work by blocking alpha receptors on the smooth muscles of blood vessels, which leads to the relaxation of these muscles. This reduces resistance in the blood vessels and lowers blood pressure.

Possible side effects:

- Dizziness or lightheadedness, primarily upon standing (orthostatic hypotension)
- Rapid or irregular heartbeat (palpitations)
- Headaches
- Fatigue
- Fluid retention, leading to swelling in the legs, ankles, or feet

Examples:

- Prazosin (Minipress)
- Terazosin (Hytrin)
- Doxazosin (Cardura)

7. Alpha-beta-blockers

Alpha-beta blockers combine the actions of alpha-blockers and beta-blockers. They block both alpha receptors and beta receptors, relaxing blood vessels and slowing down the heart rate. This dual action results in lowered blood pressure.

Possible side effects:

- Dizziness or lightheadedness, primarily upon standing (orthostatic hypotension)
- Fatigue
- Headaches
- Cold hands and feet
- Rapid or irregular heartbeat (palpitations)
- Erectile dysfunction

Examples:

- Carvedilol (Coreg)
- Labetalol (Trandate, Normodyne)

8. Central-acting agents

Central-acting agents work on the brain, reducing the signals sent to the nervous system that constrict blood vessels and increase heart rate. By decreasing these signals, these medications help lower blood pressure.

Possible side effects:

- Dizziness or lightheadedness
- Dry mouth
- Constipation
- Fatigue or drowsiness
- Erectile dysfunction

Examples:

- Clonidine (Catapres)
- Methyldopa (Aldomet)
- Guanfacine (Tenex)

9. Vasodilators

Vasodilators directly act on the smooth muscles of blood vessels, causing them to relax and widen. This dilation of blood vessels reduces resistance and lowers blood pressure.

Possible side effects:

- Headaches
- Rapid or irregular heartbeat (palpitations)
- Flushing or redness in the face
- Swelling in the legs, ankles, or feet
- Chest pain or discomfort

Examples:

- Hydralazine (Apresoline)
- Minoxidil (Loniten)

10. Aldosterone receptor antagonists

Aldosterone receptor antagonists (ARAs) are a class of medications that inhibit the action of aldosterone, a hormone that regulates salt and water balance in the body. By blocking aldosterone, ARAs promote the excretion of sodium and water and the retention of potassium, helping to reduce blood volume and lower blood pressure. This makes them valuable for managing conditions such as hypertension and heart failure. These are both part of the afore-mentioned potassium-sparing diuretics.

Possible side effects:

- Hyperkalemia (increased potassium levels in the blood)
- Gynecomastia (breast enlargement in males)
- Menstrual irregularities
- Impotence
- Kidney function abnormalities

Examples:

- Spironolactone (Aldactone)
- Eplerenone (Inspra)

11. Direct renin inhibitors

Direct renin inhibitors (DRIs) are a type of medication that works to control hypertension by directly inhibiting renin, an enzyme that triggers a sequence of reactions leading to blood vessel constriction and sodium retention. By blocking renin, these drugs help relax blood vessels and reduce fluid retention, effectively lowering blood pressure.

Possible side effects:

- Dizziness or lightheadedness
- Cough
- Diarrhea
- Flu-like symptoms
- Fatigue
- Elevated potassium levels in the blood (hyperkalemia)

Examples:

- Aliskiren (Tekturna or Rasilez)

As we've explored the different classes of blood pressure medications, it's essential to remember that each person's needs are unique. A healthcare provider can help you determine the best medication or combination of medications for your situation.

It's also crucial to communicate any side effects you experience with your healthcare provider, as they may need to adjust your treatment plan accordingly. Together, you can work toward effectively managing your high blood pressure and maintaining optimal health.

COMBINATION THERAPY

Managing high blood pressure often requires a comprehensive strategy that combines lifestyle modifications and medications. Addressing your diet, exercise, stress levels, and smoking habits can significantly impact your blood pressure and help minimize the risk of complications associated with this condition.

However, there are instances where lifestyle adjustments alone may not suffice to bring your blood pressure down to a healthy range. In such cases, medication may be necessary to assist in lowering your blood pressure.

Your healthcare provider plays a crucial role in recommending the most suitable medication or combination of medications for you. They will take into account your medical history, risk factors, and overall health status.

When it comes to treating high blood pressure, employing a combination of two or more drugs can improve both blood pressure control and tolerance to the medications. Utilizing two medications with different mechanisms of action can be more effective in lowering blood pressure compared to merely increasing the dose of a single drug.

This approach also enables the use of lower doses for each medication, which can result in fewer side effects and promote adherence to the prescribed treatment. Research has demonstrated that combination therapy can be more effective than relying on a single drug alone, helping individuals with high blood pressure to better manage their condition.

While combination therapy for high blood pressure can yield remarkable results, it is vital to collaborate closely with your healthcare provider to determine the most appropriate combination of medications tailored to your needs. It's important to note that not all medications can be safely combined, and certain combinations may lead to interactions or side effects that could be detrimental to your health.

To better understand the benefits of combination therapy, let's explore some of the reasons why it can be a more practical approach:

1. Enhanced blood pressure control

By targeting different aspects of the blood pressure regulation system, combination therapy can provide a more comprehensive approach to managing high blood pressure. For example, combining a diuretic, which removes excess fluid from the body, with a beta-blocker, which reduces the heart rate and force of contraction, can result in more effective blood pressure control than using either drug alone.

2. Minimized side effects

Since combination therapy often involves lower doses of each medication, the risk of side effects can be reduced. Lower doses also make it easier for patients to tolerate the medications, increasing the likelihood of adherence to the treatment plan.

3. Improved treatment adherence

Taking multiple medications can be challenging for some individuals, but combination therapy can simplify the process. Many pharmaceutical companies offer fixed-dose combination pills, which contain two or more blood pressure-lowering medications in a single tablet. This can make it more convenient for patients to take their medications as prescribed, improving treatment adherence and overall blood pressure control.

4. Faster blood pressure reduction

In some cases, using combination therapy can lead to a quicker reduction in blood pressure. This can be particularly beneficial for individuals with severely elevated blood pressure or those at high risk for complications related to high blood pressure.

Despite its benefits, it's essential to recognize that combination therapy is not without potential drawbacks. Some of the challenges associated with this approach include:

1. Drug interactions

Combining multiple medications increases the risk of drug interactions, which can either reduce the effectiveness of the medications or cause harmful side effects. It's crucial to discuss all medications you're taking, including over-the-counter drugs and supplements, with your healthcare provider to minimize this risk.

2. Increased cost

Using multiple medications can lead to higher treatment costs, which may be a barrier for some individuals. However, the potential for improved blood pressure control and reduced risk of complications may offset these costs in the long run.

3. Complexity of treatment

Managing multiple medications can be complex, particularly for older adults or those with cognitive impairments. It's essential to work closely with your healthcare provider and develop strategies to simplify your treatment regimen and ensure proper medication management and adherence.

To overcome these challenges, and maximize the benefits of combination therapy, consider the following strategies:

1. Open communication with your healthcare provider

Maintain an open dialogue with your healthcare provider about your symptoms, concerns, and the medications you're taking. This will enable them to better understand your unique needs and monitor your progress while adjusting your treatment plan as needed.

2. Adherence to your treatment plan

Following your prescribed treatment plan is crucial for achieving optimal blood pressure control. Remember to take your medications as directed and notify your healthcare provider if you experience any side effects or challenges with adherence.

3. Regular monitoring of blood pressure

Regularly monitoring your blood pressure, either at home or through visits to your healthcare provider, will help you and your provider assess the effectiveness of your treatment plan and make necessary adjustments. Home blood pressure monitoring can be especially helpful in identifying the impact of lifestyle modifications and medication changes on your blood pressure.

4. Lifestyle modifications

In addition to combination therapy, continue to prioritize lifestyle changes, such as healthy eating, regular exercise, stress management, and smoking cessation. These modifications can not only help lower your blood pressure but also improve your overall health and well-being.

5. Stay informed and proactive

Educate yourself about high blood pressure and the various medications used to treat it. Being informed and proactive about your health can help you make more informed decisions and engage in meaningful discussions with your healthcare provider.

In essence, combination therapy can be a highly effective approach for managing high blood pressure, particularly when paired with lifestyle modifications. By working closely with your healthcare provider, carefully monitoring your blood pressure, and adhering to your treatment plan, you can take control of your high blood pressure and work toward a healthier future.

Remember, each person's journey with high blood pressure is unique, and finding the right combination of medications and lifestyle changes may take time, but with persistence and support from your healthcare team, you can achieve better blood pressure control and improve your overall quality of life.

HYPERTENSION MEDICATION INTERACTION WITH OTC DRUGS

Hypertensive medications play a critical role in managing high blood pressure, but they can also interact with various foods, supplements, and over-the-counter (OTC) drugs. These interactions can influence the effectiveness of your blood pressure medications or heighten the risk of side effects. It's crucial to exercise caution when taking hypertension medications and to consult your healthcare provider about any potential interactions.

Your healthcare provider may suggest avoiding specific foods, supplements, or OTC drugs or modify the dosage of your medication to prevent undesired interactions. Here are some key points to consider when using hypertension medications in conjunction with OTC drugs:

1. Over-the-counter pain relievers

Nonsteroidal anti-inflammatory drugs (NSAIDs) like ibuprofen, aspirin, and naproxen are commonly used OTC pain relievers. However, these medications can reduce the effectiveness of certain blood pressure medications and even cause your blood pressure to rise. If you require a pain reliever, it's advisable to discuss the safest options with your healthcare provider, who may recommend alternatives like acetaminophen.

2. Cold and flu medications

Decongestants such as phenylephrine and pseudoephedrine are found in many cold and flu medications which can elevate your blood pressure and interfere with the effectiveness of your hypertension medications. Before taking any cold or flu remedies, consult your healthcare provider or pharmacist to ensure they are safe for you to use.

3. Herbal supplements

Some herbal supplements, such as St. John's Wort, ginkgo biloba, and ginseng, can interact with blood pressure medications, altering their effectiveness or increasing the risk of side effects. Before starting any herbal supplement, discuss your intentions with your healthcare provider, who can advise you on potential interactions and safety concerns.

4. Antacids and acid reducers

Some antacids and acid reducers, like calcium carbonate or proton pump inhibitors, can interfere with the absorption of certain blood pressure medications. If you need to take these medications, consult your healthcare provider about possible interactions and the best time to take them to minimize any adverse effects.

5. Caffeine

While it is not an OTC medication, it's essential to be mindful of your caffeine intake when taking hypertension medications. Caffeine can cause a temporary spike in blood pressure, which could counteract the effects of your medications. Monitor your caffeine consumption and discuss any concerns with your healthcare provider.

6. Alcohol

Similar to caffeine, alcohol can impact your blood pressure and interact with your hypertension medications. Excessive alcohol consumption can raise your blood pressure and reduce the effectiveness of your medications. It's crucial to limit alcohol intake and follow your healthcare provider's recommendations.

To sum it up, it's vital to be cautious and well-informed when using hypertension medications in combination with OTC drugs, supplements, or certain substances like caffeine and alcohol. Regular communication with your healthcare provider can help you navigate potential interactions, ensuring your medications are working effectively and safely.

COMMON HIGH BLOOD PRESSURE MEDICATION INTERACTIONS

High blood pressure medication interactions can occur with various substances, including food, beverages, dietary supplements, and other drugs. Understanding these interactions is essential for the safe and effective management of high blood pressure. Let's delve into some common interactions that you should be aware of:

Drugs with Food and Beverages

Certain foods and beverages can interact with high blood pressure medications, impacting their effectiveness or causing side effects. For instance:

- Grapefruit juice: This beverage can interfere with the metabolism of some calcium channel blockers, causing an increase in drug levels and potentially leading to side effects.
- Potassium-rich foods: Consuming large amounts of potassium-rich foods while taking potassium-sparing diuretics can lead to dangerously high potassium levels in the blood, which can cause heart rhythm problems.
- Alcohol: Excessive alcohol consumption can raise blood pressure and reduce the effectiveness of high blood pressure medications.

It's essential to discuss any dietary concerns with your healthcare provider to minimize potential interactions and maintain the effectiveness of your medications.

Drugs with Dietary Supplements

Dietary supplements can also interact with high blood pressure medications:

- Coenzyme Q10 (CoQ10): While CoQ10 is often used for heart health, it can interfere with the effectiveness of certain blood pressure medications, like beta-blockers and diuretics.
- St. John's Wort: This herbal supplement may interact with blood pressure medications, altering their effectiveness or increasing the risk of side effects.
- Potassium supplements: Similar to potassium-rich foods, potassium supplements can be problematic when taken with potassium-sparing diuretics, leading to dangerously high potassium levels.

Before starting any dietary supplement, consult your healthcare provider to avoid potential interactions.

Drugs with Other Drugs

High blood pressure medications can also interact with other prescription and over-the-counter drugs, including:

- **Antihistamines**: These medications, commonly used to treat allergy symptoms, can counteract the blood pressure-lowering effects of certain medications, like alpha-blockers.
- **Bronchodilators:** Asthma medications, such as albuterol, can cause an increase in heart rate and blood pressure. This may interfere with the effectiveness of your high blood pressure medications.
- **Cordarone (amiodarone):** This antiarrhythmic drug can interact with beta-blockers and calcium channel blockers, potentially causing dangerous heart rhythm disturbances.
- **Nasal decongestants**: Decongestants found in cold and allergy medications can raise blood pressure and interfere with the effectiveness of high blood pressure medications.
- **Nicotine replacement products:** Nicotine, whether from smoking or replacement products, can raise blood pressure and counteract the effects of high blood pressure medications.

To avoid harmful drug interactions, inform your healthcare provider of all medications and supplements you are taking.

In summary, it's crucial to be aware of common high blood pressure medication interactions with food, beverages, dietary supplements, and other drugs. These interactions can impact the effectiveness of your medications or increase the risk of side effects.

By discussing potential interactions with your healthcare provider and following their guidance, you can safely manage your high blood pressure and avoid complications. Stay informed, be proactive, and maintain open communication with your healthcare team to ensure the best possible outcomes in your high blood pressure management journey.

TIPS TO AVOID INTERACTIONS

To avoid interactions between high blood pressure medications and other substances, it's essential to take proactive steps and maintain open communication with your healthcare team. Here are some practical tips to help minimize potential interactions and ensure the safe and effective management of your high blood pressure:

1. Ensure all your healthcare providers are aware of all the medicines you are taking, including prescription drugs, over-the-counter medications, dietary and herbal supplements, and vitamins. This will enable them to better evaluate any potential interactions and recommend suitable treatments.
2. Before taking any new medication, consult your healthcare provider or pharmacist and ask essential questions, such as whether the new drug will interact

with your current medications, the best time to take it, and possible side effects.
3. Drug interaction checkers, available online or as mobile apps, can help you identify potential interactions between your medications. While these tools can be helpful, they should not replace professional advice from your healthcare provider.
4. Carefully read the labels of all over-the-counter and prescription medications you take. Labels often contain crucial information about potential interactions and side effects.
5. By using one pharmacy for all your prescriptions, you can ensure that the pharmacist has a complete record of your medications, making it easier for them to identify potential interactions and provide personalized guidance.

Remember, managing high blood pressure is an ongoing process, and it's crucial to stay informed, proactive, and engaged in your treatment plan. With the support of your healthcare team and the adoption of these practical tips, you can achieve better blood pressure control and enjoy a healthier future.

QUESTIONS TO ASK YOUR HEALTHCARE PROVIDER

Before starting any medication for high blood pressure, it's essential to have an open and thorough conversation with your healthcare provider to ensure the chosen medication is both safe and effective for your specific needs. To help guide your discussion, here are ten important questions you should consider asking your doctor or pharmacist:

1. What is the primary function of this medication?

Ask your healthcare provider about the intended purpose of the medication, how it works, and the expected benefits for your blood pressure management.

2. How and when should I take this medication?

Inquire about the appropriate dosage, timing, and whether the medication should be taken with or without food. This information is crucial to ensure proper absorption and effectiveness.

3. Can I take this medication with other drugs?

Discuss potential interactions with other medications you are currently taking and learn about any warning signs of adverse drug interactions.

4. Are there possible side effects or interactions with food or supplements?

Understand the potential side effects and any interactions with specific foods, beverages, or dietary supplements that could affect the medication's effectiveness or safety.

5. How long will it take before the medication begins to work?

Ask your healthcare provider about the expected time frame for the medication to start showing its effects on your blood pressure.

6. How can I determine if the medication is working, and how frequently should I monitor my blood pressure?

Learn how to evaluate the effectiveness of your medication and the recommended frequency for blood pressure monitoring.

7. Are there any lifestyle changes I should make while taking this medication?

Discuss any recommended adjustments to your diet, exercise routine, or other lifestyle factors that may complement your high blood pressure treatment plan.

8. What precautions should I take while on this medication?

Understand any specific precautions you should be aware of while taking the medication, such as avoiding particular activities, foods, or beverages.

9. What should I do if I miss a dose or accidentally take too much medication?

Learn the appropriate steps to take in case you miss a dose or accidentally take more medication than prescribed.

10. When should I schedule a follow-up appointment to assess my blood pressure and evaluate the medication's effectiveness?

Determine the optimal time for a follow-up appointment to review your blood pressure levels and discuss the medication's effectiveness with your healthcare provider.

By asking these vital questions and staying informed about your medication and its potential interactions, you can better manage your high blood pressure and reduce the risk of complications. Remember, active involvement in your treatment plan and open communication with your healthcare team is key to achieving optimal blood pressure control and improving your overall health.

As we wrap up this chapter, I hope I've been able to provide you with a solid understanding of the different medications available for managing high blood pressure and the crucial steps to avoid harmful drug interactions. Remember, knowledge and communication are key to ensuring the safe and effective use of these medications.

In the upcoming chapter, we'll dive into the world of dietary modifications and explore various ways to effectively and safely lower your blood pressure through changes in your eating habits. This valuable information can make a significant difference in your blood pressure management journey.

4

HEALTHY FOOD FOR A HAPPY HEART

As we unveil the secrets to a rejuvenated life in this chapter, you'll discover transformative diet modifications to safely reduce blood pressure and enhance overall well-being. In Jim Rohn's words: *"Take care of your body. It's the only place you have to live."* After all, keeping yourself well informed about your health and actively pursuing lifestyle adjustment knowledge is imperative.

Another measure to enhance your well-being is to ultimately become your own strongest supporter. Minor changes to your everyday habits, like incorporating consistent physical activity, embracing a nutritious diet, and regulating stress levels, can decrease your blood pressure and diminish the risks linked to hypertension.

YOUR DIET AND HEART HEALTH: A CRUCIAL CONNECTION

The food choices we make significantly impact our heart health. By embracing diets that promote cardiovascular well-being, we can lower the risk of heart disease. One such diet is the DASH (Dietary Approaches to Stop Hypertension) diet.

THE DASH DIET: A LIFELINE FOR YOUR HEART

The DASH diet is nutrient-rich and designed to lower blood pressure and protect your heart. Focusing on consuming whole foods encourages a balanced intake of fruits, vegetables, whole grains, lean proteins, and low-fat dairy products.

Potential Benefits of the DASH Diet

Adopting the DASH diet may reduce blood pressure, improve cholesterol levels, and decrease the risk of heart disease and stroke. It can also promote weight loss and support overall health.

DASH Diet Suitability

While the DASH diet is generally beneficial, individual results may vary. Consulting a healthcare professional is recommended to determine if it's the right fit for your unique health needs.

Salt Restriction: Striking the Right Balance

Excess salt consumption can contribute to high blood pressure, but overly restricting salt may negatively affect the body's sodium balance. Finding a moderate approach is essential, following recommended daily intake guidelines.

DASH Diet Foods: Dos and Don'ts

Enjoy Fruits, vegetables, whole grains, lean meats, fish, poultry, nuts, seeds, legumes, and low-fat dairy products. Avoid Processed foods, high-sodium items, saturated fats, sugary beverages, and excessive alcohol.

Sample Menu

A well-planned DASH diet menu incorporates a variety of whole foods, providing diverse flavors and nutrients. A sample week might include whole-grain oatmeal with berries, grilled chicken salads, brown rice with steamed vegetables, and baked fish with quinoa.

▷ *Day 1: Menu*

Breakfast

- 1 cup of oatmeal without salt
- 1/4 cup raisins
- 1 medium banana
- 1 cup fat-free milk
- Coffee, tea, or water

Lunch

- Hummus plate with:

  - 1/2 cup hummus
  - 1/2 medium red pepper
  - 1/2 medium cucumber
  - 10 baby carrots
  - 1 whole-grain pita pocket

- Water

Dinner

- Roasted salmon with:

  - 4 ounces of salmon
  - Maple balsamic glaze

- 1 cup whole-grain and wild rice blend
- 3/4 cup green beans with red bell peppers
- 1/2 cup canned pear slices in juice
- Tea, hot or cold, and not sweetened

Snack (anytime)

- 1 cup low-fat yogurt
- 1 medium peach

▷ *Day 2: Menu*

Breakfast

- 1 cup mixed fruit such as melon and grapes
- 1/2 whole-wheat bagel
- 1 tablespoon natural peanut butter
- 1 cup skim milk
- Coffee, tea, or water.

Lunch

- Spinach salad with:

  - 3 cups fresh spinach leaves
  - 1 sliced pear
  - 1/2 cup canned mandarin oranges
  - 1 tablespoon red wine vinegar

- 1 tablespoon olive oil
- 1 ounce of goat cheese
- 3 ounces of cooked chicken

- 1 small whole-wheat roll
- Water

Dinner

- Vegetarian pasta with:

  - 1/2 cup marinara sauce
  - 1 cup chopped summer squash
  - 1/2 cup frozen chopped spinach
  - 1 1/2 cups whole-wheat pasta

- 1 cup melon
- 1 cup skim milk

Snack (anytime)

- 1/4 cup trail mix, not salted

▷ *Day 3: Menu*

Breakfast

- 1 cup mixed fruit such as melon and grapes

- 1/2 whole-wheat bagel
- 1 tablespoon natural peanut butter
- 1 cup skim milk
- Coffee, tea, or water.

Lunch

- Spinach salad with:

  - 3 cups fresh spinach leaves
  - 1 sliced pear
  - 1/2 cup canned mandarin oranges
  - 1 tablespoon red wine vinegar
  - 1 tablespoon olive oil
  - 1 ounce of goat cheese
  - 3 ounces of cooked chicken

- 1 small whole-wheat roll
- Water

Dinner

- Vegetarian pasta with:

  - 1/2 cup marinara sauce
  - 1 cup chopped summer squash
  - 1/2 cup frozen chopped spinach
  - 1 1/2 cups whole-wheat pasta

- 1 cup melon
- 1 cup skim milk

Snack (anytime)

- 1/4 cup trail mix, not salted

Adjusting Your Diet to DASH Guidelines

Follow DASH guidelines, prioritize whole foods, control portion sizes, and minimize processed items. Gradually increase your intake of fruits, vegetables, and whole grains, while reducing saturated fats, sodium, and added sugars. Remember, small changes can make a significant impact on your heart health.

Embracing the DASH Lifestyle: Tips and Strategies

1. **Gradual Change:** Instead of overhauling your diet overnight, make incremental adjustments to ensure a smoother, sustainable transition. This approach can help you adapt to the DASH diet without feeling overwhelmed.
2. **Meal Planning**: Create weekly meal plans to streamline grocery shopping and avoid impulsive, unhealthy food choices. This strategy can save time, reduce stress, and ensure you stay on track with your DASH diet goals.

3. **Mindful Eating:** Pay attention to hunger and satiety cues and savor each bite. By eating slowly and deliberately, you can improve digestion, enjoy your food more, and prevent overeating.
4. **Home Cooking:** Prepare meals at home to control the ingredients and cooking methods, ensuring that your dishes align with DASH guidelines. Experiment with new recipes, flavors, and techniques to keep your meals exciting and satisfying.
5. **Hydration:** Drinking water is essential for overall health and can help with weight management. Stay hydrated by consuming water throughout the day, replacing sugary beverages with healthier alternatives like herbal tea or infused water.
6. **Support System:** Engage with friends or family members who share your health goals or join online communities centered around the DASH diet. A strong support network can provide encouragement, motivation, and accountability.
7. **Regular Check-Ins**: Monitor your progress by checking blood pressure, weight, and other health indicators. This practice will help you evaluate the effectiveness of the DASH diet and make any necessary adjustments.

Remember, the journey to a healthier heart begins with a single step. Embrace the DASH diet and its principles, and you'll be well on your way to improved cardiovascular health and overall well-being.

THE MEDITERRANEAN DIET: A JOURNEY TO WHOLESOME WELLNESS

The Mediterranean diet is a heart-healthy eating plan inspired by the traditional cuisine of countries bordering the Mediterranean Sea. It emphasizes plant-based foods, healthy fats, and moderate protein consumption, focusing on quality, variety, and balance.

Potential Benefits of the Mediterranean Diet

Adopting this diet may improve cardiovascular health, weight loss, better blood sugar control, and reduce risk of chronic diseases. Its nutrient-dense, antioxidant-rich nature also supports overall well-being and longevity.

Embarking on the Mediterranean Path

To start, gradually incorporate the dietary principles and food choices typical of the Mediterranean lifestyle. Choose whole, minimally processed foods, and explore new flavors and cooking techniques inspired by Mediterranean cuisine.

Foods to Savor

Enjoy a diverse range of plant-based foods like fruits, vegetables, whole grains, nuts, seeds, and legumes. Choose healthy fats such as olive oil, avocados, and fatty fish like salmon and sardines. Consume moderate amounts of lean proteins, including poultry, eggs, and dairy products.

Foods to Limit

Minimize the intake of red meat, processed foods, refined sugars, and unhealthy fats like trans fats and saturated fats. Consume alcohol, particularly red wine, in moderation.

Sample Weekly Menu

A well-crafted Mediterranean diet menu is rich in flavors, colors, and textures. A sample week might include whole-grain salads with fresh vegetables and herbs, grilled fish drizzled with olive oil, lentil soup, vegetable-stuffed peppers, and fresh fruit with yogurt for dessert. Embrace the Mediterranean diet to nourish your body with wholesome, delicious meals, and embark on a journey to enhanced health, vitality, and longevity.

▷ **Monday**

- Breakfast: Greek yogurt with strawberries and chia seeds
- Lunch: A whole-grain sandwich with hummus and vegetables
- Dinner: A tuna salad with greens and olive oil, as well as a fruit salad

▷ **Tuesday**

- Breakfast: Oatmeal with blueberries
- Lunch: Caprese zucchini noodles with mozzarella, cherry tomatoes, olive oil, and balsamic vinegar
- Dinner: A salad with tomatoes, olives, cucumbers, farro, baked trout, and feta cheese

▷ **Wednesday**

- Breakfast: An omelet with mushrooms, tomatoes, and onions
- Lunch: A whole-grain sandwich with cheese and fresh vegetables
- Dinner: Mediterranean lasagna

▷ **Thursday**

- Breakfast: Yogurt with sliced fruit and nuts

- Lunch: A quinoa salad with chickpeas
- Dinner: Broiled salmon with brown rice and vegetables

▷ **Friday**

- Breakfast: Eggs and sautéed vegetables with whole-wheat toast
- Lunch: Stuffed zucchini boats with pesto, turkey sausage, tomatoes, bell peppers, and cheese
- Dinner: Grilled lamb with salad and baked potato

▷ **Saturday**

- Breakfast: Oatmeal with nuts and raisins or apple slices
- Lunch: Lentil salad with feta, tomatoes, cucumbers, and olives
- Dinner: Mediterranean pizza made with whole-wheat pita bread and topped with cheese, vegetables, and olives

▷ **Sunday**

- Breakfast: An omelet with veggies and olives
- Lunch: Bowl with feta, onions, tomatoes, hummus, and rice

- Dinner: Grilled chicken with vegetables, sweet potato fries, and fresh fruit

There's usually no need to count calories or track macronutrients (protein, fat, and carbs) on the Mediterranean diet unless you are managing your glucose levels. It is essential to consume all foods in moderation and not overindulge.

DIETARY WISDOM FOR A HEALTHY HEART: PRACTICAL TIPS AND TRICKS

Caring for your heart is paramount, and the choices you make at the dining table play a crucial role in safeguarding your cardiovascular well-being. Here are some essential diet tips to help you maintain a healthy heart:

1. Portion Control: Master the Art

Overeating can lead to weight gain, increasing the risk of heart disease. Learning to control portion sizes is key to maintaining a healthy weight and reducing cardiovascular strain. Use smaller plates, check serving sizes on food labels, and listen to your body's hunger and satiety cues to avoid overindulging.

2. A Colorful Plate: Embrace Vegetables and Fruits

Vegetables and fruits are abundant in vitamins, minerals, fiber, and antioxidants that support heart health. Aim to fill half of your plate with a colorful variety of these nutrient powerhouses. Incorporate them into your meals as salads, side dishes, or even as healthy snacks between meals.

3. The Wholesome Choice: Choose Whole Grains

Whole grains, such as brown rice, quinoa, oats, and whole wheat, are rich in fiber and essential nutrients that help regulate blood pressure and cholesterol levels. Replace refined grains with whole-grain options to enhance heart health and maintain steady blood sugar levels.

4. Fats: Discerning the Good from the Bad

Not all fats are created equal. Prioritize heart-healthy fats, like those found in olive oil, nuts, seeds, and avocados, while limiting unhealthy fats, such as trans fats and saturated fats found in processed and fried foods. Moderation is key, even with healthy fats, as they are calorie-dense.

5. Protein Power: Lean and Low-Fat

Choose low-fat protein sources, such as lean meats, poultry, fish, beans, legumes, and low-fat dairy products. Fish, particularly fatty varieties like salmon and mackerel, are rich in omega-3 fatty acids that promote heart health. Aim to incorporate at least two servings of fish per week.

6. Sodium Savvy: Tread Lightly on Salt

Excessive sodium intake can elevate blood pressure, increasing the risk of heart disease. Limit processed foods, which are often high in salt, and season your meals with herbs, spices, and other low-sodium flavor enhancers. Aim to stay within the recommended daily sodium intake guidelines.

7. Planning for Success: Crafting Daily Menus

Planning your meals in advance enables you to make healthier choices and avoid impulsive, less nutritious options. Create a balanced menu that incorporates heart-healthy foods and allows for some flexibility. A well-planned menu helps you stay on track with your dietary goals and streamlines meal preparation.

8. Indulge Mindfully: The Joy of Occasional Treats

A heart-healthy diet doesn't mean completely depriving yourself of the foods you love. Allowing yourself an occasional treat can prevent feelings of deprivation and help you stay committed to your healthy eating habits. Enjoy these indulgences mindfully and in moderation.

By incorporating these practical tips into your daily life, you can cultivate a heart-healthy diet that not only supports your cardiovascular system but also enhances your overall well-being. Remember, every small change adds up to make a significant impact on your health.

What about caffeine?

Caffeine, a naturally occurring stimulant found in coffee, has become an integral part of many people's daily routines. However, its effects on blood pressure have raised concerns, especially for individuals with hypertension. Let's delve into the connection between caffeine and blood pressure.

1. Coffee's Pressure Push: The Mechanics

Caffeine can cause a temporary increase in blood pressure by stimulating the release of stress hormones, such as adrenaline, which in turn constrict blood vessels and raise the heart rate. The exact duration and magnitude of this effect may vary based on individual factors like genetics, tolerance, and caffeine sensitivity.

2. The Long Haul: Prolonged Coffee Consumption

While the short-term effects of caffeine on blood pressure are well established, the long-term impact is less clear. Some studies suggest that regular coffee consumption may be associated with a slightly increased risk of developing hypertension, while others indicate that the body can develop a tolerance to these effects over time. More research is needed to fully understand the long-term implications of habitual coffee drinking.

3. Hypertension and Coffee: Navigating the Dilemma

For those with hypertension, it is crucial to monitor and manage blood pressure. While there is no one-size-fits-all answer, individuals with high blood pressure should consider their unique circumstances when deciding on coffee consumption.

Some may be more sensitive to caffeine's effects and should limit their intake, while others might experience little to no impact on their blood pressure. Consulting with a healthcare professional is recommended to determine the best course of action.

4. Decaf Dynamics: A Milder Jolt

Decaffeinated coffee contains only a fraction of the caffeine found in regular coffee, making it a viable alternative for those looking to minimize caffeine's effects on blood pressure. However, even decaf coffee may still cause a slight, short-lived increase in blood pressure for some individuals. Paying attention to your body's response is essential in determining whether decaf coffee is a suitable option.

5. Time to Pause: Ceasing Coffee Consumption

If you find that coffee consumption significantly raises your blood pressure or exacerbates hypertension, it may be time to consider reducing or stopping your intake. Gradually decreasing your coffee consumption can help prevent withdrawal symptoms such as headaches, fatigue, and irritability.

6. Beyond the Bean: Coffee Alternatives

For those looking to reduce or eliminate coffee consumption, several alternatives can provide a comforting ritual without blood pressure concerns. Herbal teas, like chamomile or peppermint, offer warmth and flavor without caffeine.

Green tea, while still containing some caffeine, has a lower amount than coffee and provides antioxidants that promote health. Chicory root coffee, a caffeine-free option, mimics the taste and aroma of coffee and can be a satisfying substitute.

Understanding the relationship between caffeine and blood pressure is essential for making informed decisions about your coffee consumption. Listen to your body, consult with a healthcare professional, and explore alternatives to find the right balance for your health and well-being.

7. Caffeine in Perspective: A Holistic Approach

When assessing the effects of caffeine on blood pressure, it's important to consider the broader context of your lifestyle and overall health. Factors such as diet, exercise, stress management, and sleep quality all play a significant role in determining your blood pressure and heart health.

8. Mindful Consumption: Know Your Limits

Being aware of your personal caffeine tolerance and sensitivity can help you make more informed choices about coffee consumption. Pay attention to how your body reacts to caffeine and adjust your intake accordingly. It is generally recommended not to exceed 400 mg of caffeine per day, which is roughly equivalent to four 8-ounce cups of brewed coffee.

9. Caffeine and Beyond Coffee's Nutrient Profile

While the focus is often on caffeine's impact on blood pressure, it's essential to recognize that coffee also contains various beneficial compounds, including antioxidants and polyphenols. These bioactive compounds can help reduce inflammation, protect against cellular damage, and support overall health. Moderation is key—enjoy the potential benefits without overdoing it.

10. Caffeine and Lifestyle: Striking a Balance

When looking to manage blood pressure and maintain heart health, a comprehensive approach that encompasses various aspects of your lifestyle is crucial. In addition to monitoring your caffeine intake, focus on eating a balanced diet rich in whole foods, engaging in regular physical activity, managing stress through techniques like meditation or yoga, and getting adequate, restful sleep.

Navigating the complex relationship between caffeine and blood pressure requires self-awareness, knowledge, and adaptability. By incorporating a holistic approach to your health and considering your unique circumstances, you can make well-informed decisions about coffee consumption that support your overall well-being and heart health. Embrace a balanced lifestyle and enjoy your coffee—or alternatives—mindfully and responsibly.

HEART-HEALTHY PANTRY: 21 FOODS TO NOURISH AND PROTECT YOUR HEART

1. **Fresh Herbs:** Flavorful alternatives to salt, these aromatic plants help reduce sodium intake and support heart health.
2. **Black Beans:** Rich in fiber and protein, these legumes lower cholesterol and maintain stable blood sugar levels.
3. **Red Wine and Resveratrol:** Moderate consumption of red wine, containing the antioxidant resveratrol, may protect against heart disease.
4. **Salmon:** This superfood is packed with omega-3 fatty acids, which decrease inflammation and improve cardiovascular function.
5. **Tuna:** Another excellent source of omega-3s, tuna supports heart health and reduces inflammation.
6. **Olive Oil:** Rich in heart-healthy monounsaturated fats, olive oil can help lower bad cholesterol and reduce the risk of heart disease.
7. **Walnuts:** These nuts provide essential nutrients, including omega-3s, antioxidants, and fiber, promoting a healthy heart.
8. **Almonds:** High in monounsaturated fats, almonds help lower cholesterol levels and improve heart health.
9. **Edamame:** Soybeans are a great source of plant-based protein, fiber, and heart-healthy nutrients.

10. **Tofu:** Another soy-based option, tofu is low in saturated fat and high in nutrients, supporting heart health.
11. **Sweet Potatoes:** Packed with vitamins, minerals, and fiber, these tubers help regulate blood pressure and maintain heart health.
12. **Oranges:** Rich in potassium and vitamin C, oranges support healthy blood pressure and protect the cardiovascular system.
13. **Swiss Chard:** This leafy green is high in magnesium and potassium, essential minerals for heart health.
14. **Barley:** A whole grain containing soluble fiber, barley helps lower cholesterol and supports cardiovascular well-being.
15. **Oatmeal:** Rich in fiber and nutrients, oatmeal reduces cholesterol levels and improves heart health.
16. **Flaxseed:** A plant-based source of omega-3 fatty acids, flaxseed promotes heart health and reduces inflammation.
17. **Low-Fat Yogurt:** A probiotic-rich source of calcium and protein, low-fat yogurt supports a healthy heart.
18. **Foods Fortified with Sterols:** These plant compounds help lower cholesterol levels, promoting heart health.
19. **Cherries:** With anti-inflammatory and antioxidant properties, cherries help protect the heart.
20. **Blueberries:** Packed with antioxidants, these berries support heart health and reduce inflammation.

21. **Dark Leafy Greens:** Nutrient-dense and rich in antioxidants, leafy greens like spinach and kale contribute to a healthy heart.

Incorporate these 21 heart-healthy foods into your diet to nourish and protect your cardiovascular system, promoting overall well-being. Altering your dietary habits can significantly contribute to reducing your blood pressure.

However, it is essential to remember that a comprehensive approach to managing high blood pressure also involves exercise and weight management. In the next chapter, we will explore the vital roles that physical activity and sustaining a healthy weight play in safely and effectively lowering your blood pressure. By doing so, you can decrease your chances of developing heart disease and enhance your general well-being. It's time to embrace an active lifestyle and embark on the journey toward optimal health!

5

MOVE IT AND LOSE IT

"Even when all is known, the care of a man is not yet complete because eating alone will not keep a man well; he must also exercise. While possessing opposite qualities, food, and exercise work together to produce health."

— HIPPOCRATES

These wise words from the "Father of Medicine" himself emphasize a profound truth about our well-being: our health journey is an intricate dance between diet and exercise. I'll tell you why.

Imagine your body as an engine, fueled by the food you eat, and exercise acts as the perfect catalyst, enhancing the efficiency of this engine. This chapter explores this interplay, focusing on the pivotal role of physical exercise and weight management in lowering blood pressure and ameliorating heart health.

This chapter will dive deep into the connection between our bodies' physical exertion and heart health. We'll explore how different forms of exercise contribute to weight management and, consequently, blood pressure control.

GET MOVING

There is an old saying: "A body in motion stays in motion." This principle couldn't be truer when managing high blood pressure. Regular physical activity is not just a recommendation but a necessity, acting as an antidote to hypertension and an elixir for overall heart health. But how does exercise do this?

Exercise aids in lowering blood pressure by enhancing cardiovascular health and boosting the efficiency of our circulatory system. As we move, our heart, the hard-working muscle that it is pumps blood throughout our body more effectively. This efficiency reduces the force on our artery walls, thereby decreasing our blood pressure. It's a simple yet powerful cycle that starts with the decision to get moving.

As we maintain a healthy weight, our blood pressure levels tend to normalize, reducing the likelihood of hypertension and associated health risks. Furthermore, physical activity helps manage other risk factors synonymous with high blood pressure. Take obesity, for example. Regular exercise aids in weight management, reducing the strain on the heart that excess weight often causes.

For those battling diabetes, another risk factor for high blood pressure, exercise is a vital ally. Physical activity aids in regulating blood sugar levels, increasing insulin sensitivity, and promoting a healthier metabolic state. By integrating regular exercise into our routine, we can manage diabetes more effectively, mitigating its impact on our blood pressure.

Stress, a silent contributor to high blood pressure, can be significantly managed through regular exercise. Physical activity releases endorphins, the body's natural mood lifters, promoting well-being and relaxation. This stress reduction can indirectly aid blood pressure control, contributing to our overall heart health.

Now, let's dive into the benefits of exercise on heart health. Regular physical activity strengthens the heart muscle, enabling it to pump blood more efficiently, thereby reducing the pressure on the arteries. This heart-strengthening effect, over time, can lead to a sustainable decrease in resting heart rate and blood pressure.

Exercise also promotes better lipid profiles by raising good cholesterol (HDL) levels and reducing bad cholesterol (LDL) levels. This balance can prevent cholesterol buildup in arteries, reducing the risk of atherosclerosis and heart disease.

Moreover, the increased blood flow during exercise delivers more oxygen and essential nutrients to the tissues, including the heart. This enhanced circulation promotes the healing and growth of the cells, further improving the function and structure of the cardiovascular system.

Physical activity also aids in maintaining a healthy vascular function by improving endothelial function, promoting vascular remodeling, and enhancing baroreflex sensitivity. These changes can further lower blood pressure and contribute to the heart's overall health.

Moreover, when safeguarding heart health, physical activity wears the crown. Its benefits extend far beyond calorie-burning or physique-shaping; it is the linchpin in maintaining optimal cardiovascular health. But what makes regular exercise such a powerful ally for our hearts?

1. The heart is a muscle; like other muscles, it grows stronger with exercise. Regular physical activity enables our heart to pump blood more efficiently throughout the body, reducing the strain on this vital organ. Over time, this lessens the risk of heart disease, including conditions like heart failure.
2. Exercise positively influences blood flow in multiple ways. It helps arteries maintain their elasticity, ensuring smooth, unimpeded blood flow. Enhanced

circulation also means more oxygen and vital nutrients are delivered to the body's tissues, leading to better overall health and, specifically, a healthier heart.
3. Regular physical activity helps manage blood lipid levels, namely triglycerides, and cholesterol.
4. Exercise plays a vital role in achieving and maintaining a healthy weight, which is crucial for heart health. Excess weight strains the heart, increasing the risk of hypertension, high cholesterol, and diabetes—all risk factors for heart disease.
5. Regular physical activity helps lower blood pressure, a key benefit for those with hypertension. The heart-friendly effects of exercise extend beyond the workout period, with blood pressure often remaining lower for several hours post-exercise.
6. Exercise is an effective stressbuster. It stimulates the production of endorphins, the body's natural mood lifters. Less stress translates to lower blood pressure over time, further reducing the risk of heart disease.
7. Regular physical activity improves the body's sensitivity to insulin, reducing the risk of type 2 diabetes—a significant risk factor for heart disease. For those already living with diabetes, exercise helps manage the condition, lessening its impact on heart health.

In essence, the relationship between regular exercise and heart health is symbiotic. Physical activity nourishes our heart, providing the support it needs to function optimally, while our heart, in turn, fuels our ability to stay active, fit, and healthy. It's a beautiful, beneficial cycle, and investment in exercise truly is an investment in a healthier, heart-happy future.

EXERCISE OPTIONS FOR YOU

When it comes to exercise's beneficial effects on blood pressure, patience, and consistency are essential. It typically takes between one to three months of regular exercise to see a tangible impact on blood pressure levels. And these benefits, just like the blooms of a well-tended garden, persist only as long as you continue your exercise regimen.

But what type of exercise works best? Here's the good news: you have options, and they're all advantageous in their own unique ways.

1. *Cardiovascular or Aerobic Exercise*

This form of exercise, which includes activities like jogging, cycling, swimming, or even brisk walking, primarily targets your heart and lungs. Regular aerobic exercise strengthens your heart, making it more efficient at pumping blood and supplying your body with the oxygen it needs. This helps lower blood pressure and is excellent for overall cardiovascular health.

2. Strength Training

Lifting weights or using resistance bands are examples of strength training. While it might seem more suited for those looking to build muscle, it plays a pivotal role in heart health too. Regular strength training helps reduce body fat, increase lean muscle mass, and burn calories more efficiently. This, in turn, aids in weight management, a key factor in maintaining healthy blood pressure levels.

3. Resistance Training

Like strength training, it involves using weights or resistance bands. However, it also includes exercises that use your body weight (like push-ups or squats). This form of exercise not only builds strength and burns calories, but it can also help improve your resting metabolic rate, aiding in weight control and hence, blood pressure management.

4. Stretching

While stretching may not directly lower blood pressure, it plays a supporting role in your overall exercise regimen. Regular stretching keeps your body flexible and injury-free, allowing you to maintain a consistent exercise routine.

Furthermore, practices such as yoga, which include an emphasis on deep breathing and relaxation, can help lower stress levels, a contributing factor to high blood pressure.

Remember, a well-rounded exercise routine comprising cardiovascular exercise, strength training, resistance training, and stretching is the secret recipe to combat high blood pressure and enhance heart health. The key is to remain consistent, as the fruits of your efforts, although not immediate, will surely be rewarding. Your journey toward a healthier heart is a marathon, not a sprint.

THE ART OF EXERCISING RIGHT

When it comes to exercise, it's not merely about doing it; it's about doing it right. The duration, intensity, and consistency of your exercise routine play pivotal roles in effectively managing blood pressure and promoting overall heart health.

Let's dive into the optimal exercise framework, one that is both beneficial and sustainable.

1. *The Gold Standard – 30 Minutes of Moderate Activity*

Whether you enjoy brisk walking, a leisurely bike ride, or a spirited dance class, engaging in moderate activity for at least 30 minutes five days a week lays the foundation for a heart-healthy exercise routine. This goal is as pragmatic as it is beneficial, designed to accommodate the busiest of schedules.

2. Short on Time? Intensify!

When time constraints challenge your commitment, don't despair! The beauty of exercise lies in its flexibility. If carving out 30 minutes proves difficult, consider vigorous activities like jogging or high-intensity interval training (HIIT). A focused 20-minute session of such vigorous exercise, three to four days a week, can yield the same heart health benefits as longer, moderate activity sessions.

3. Begin at the Beginning – Gradual Is Good

If you're at the start of your exercise journey, take heart in knowing that every journey begins with a single step. Aim for consistency over intensity initially. Gradually work up to the recommended amount of exercise over a few weeks, respecting your body's pace and limitations.

4. Warming Up – The Prelude to a Safe Workout

A safe and effective workout begins with a warm-up. Consider it the gentle wake-up call that prepares your body for the activity ahead. Start with a 5- to 10-minute warm-up routine that slowly increases your heart rate while loosening your muscles and joints. The key is to increase the intensity gradually; a good gauge is being able to carry on with a conversation while exercising.

5. Cooling Down – An Essential Encore

Exercise is a cycle, and its completion lies in a proper cool-down period. After a workout, take a few minutes to slow down your activity level gradually. This wind-down phase is especially important for individuals with high blood pressure. It allows the heart rate and blood pressure to return to resting levels gradually, reducing strain on the heart.

Ultimately, the perfect exercise routine fits seamlessly into your lifestyle, is enjoyable, and respects your body's needs and limitations. Remember that the true value of exercise lies in its regularity rather than intensity. And like any good habit, the benefits of exercise compound over time. Your commitment today, however small it might seem, is an investment in a healthier, heart-happier future.

STAYING THE COURSE: NURTURING A SUSTAINABLE EXERCISE ROUTINE

Sustaining an exercise routine can be a challenge, especially in our ever-busy lives. Yet, consistency is the lifeblood of a beneficial workout regime. Here are some strategies to help you keep that commitment to your heart's health:

1. Choose an exercise activity that you enjoy. This isn't merely about 'getting fit'; it's about finding joy in movement and creating a space in your day that you look forward to. Whether it's the peace of yoga, the rhythm of dance, or the exhilaration of cycling, make sure it's something that speaks to your spirit.
2. Set realistic, achievable fitness goals. While the overarching goal is heart health, having smaller, measurable objectives can be incredibly motivating. It could be walking an extra kilometer, shaving a minute off your run time, or mastering a new yoga pose. Celebrate these milestones; they are steps on your journey to heart health.
3. Establishing a regular exercise schedule helps transform your workout from a 'to-do' into a habit. If you're a morning person, harness that energy into an invigorating start to your day. If evenings are your time, wind down with a calming yoga session. Find a rhythm that fits your lifestyle.
4. On days when time is scarce, or energy levels are low, remember that a shorter workout is better than no workout at all. Even a brisk 10-minute walk contributes to your goal. Consistency trumps duration.
5. Engage in physical activities with a partner or a group. Exercising with others can be fun and motivating. It creates a sense of community and accountability, which can help keep you on track.

6. Incorporate variety into your routine to prevent boredom. Try new activities, alternate between different types of exercises, or change your workout environment. Variety keeps your workouts fresh and exciting.
7. Rest when you need to, modify exercises when necessary, and seek professional advice if you have any health concerns. An exercise routine should respect your body's needs and limitations.

Remember, exercise is a celebration of what your body can do, not a punishment for what you eat. Let this perspective guide you in nurturing an exercise routine that enhances not only your heart health but also your overall well-being.

EXERCISE GUIDELINES FOR OLDER ADULTS

Throughout the different stages of life, our bodies undergo a variety of changes. Yet, one constant remains—the importance of physical activity. Regardless of age, exercise plays a vital role in maintaining our health and well-being. However, as we grow older, the approach to fitness necessitates more caution and care, as personal health conditions and capabilities must be prioritized.

Older adults are recommended to engage in at least 150 minutes of moderate-intensity aerobic activity per week, or 75 minutes of vigorous-intensity activity, along with muscle-strengthening activities at least twice weekly. But remember, these are general guidelines and must be adjusted to individual capacities and health circumstances.

Consultation with a healthcare provider can help design an exercise regimen that respects your specific considerations while optimizing your heart health and overall well-being. For older adults commencing their journey into regular physical activity, the best advice is to start slow. Initiating your fitness regime with low-impact activities like walking is an excellent choice.

Over time, intensity and duration can be gradually increased. Include exercises that promote flexibility, balance, and strength, such as gentle yoga or tai chi in your regimen. Most importantly, listen to your body and remember to rest when required.

Prior to starting or modifying an exercise routine, it's crucial to engage in a detailed conversation with your healthcare provider. Four essential questions should guide this discussion:

1. "What types of exercises would be suitable for me?"

Rationale: This question helps determine what forms of exercise align with your current health status, fitness level, and personal preferences. Everyone is unique, and what works well for one person may not work as well for another. Your healthcare provider can assess your current physical condition and recommend exercises that suit your fitness level. For example, if you have joint problems, low-impact exercises like swimming or cycling might be suitable.

2. "Are there any exercises or activities I should avoid?"

Rationale: Certain health conditions can make specific exercises risky. It's essential to identify these potential issues to prevent unnecessary harm and complications. Depending on your health status, your healthcare provider might advise against certain high-impact or strenuous exercises. For instance, individuals with heart conditions might need to avoid overly intense cardio workouts.

3. "How does my health condition affect my ability to exercise?"

Rationale: Your overall health and any pre-existing conditions can directly influence your capacity to exercise. Certain diseases require particular care and precautions during physical activity. For example, if you have osteoporosis, weight-bearing exercises might be beneficial, but with caution to avoid fractures. If you have diabetes, your provider will advise you on managing blood sugar levels during and after exercise.

4. "Is my preventive care up to date?"

Rationale: Keeping your preventive care up to date ensures you're exercising with the knowledge that any underlying health issues are managed and you're not putting your health at unnecessary risk. Your provider can guide you on any necessary screenings, tests, or vaccinations. For example, if you're at risk for heart disease, regular cholesterol and blood pressure check-ups are crucial.

Remember, these answers should act as a guide, and you should always consult with your healthcare provider for personalized advice. In all scenarios, the primary goal is to engage in physical activity safely and effectively for the betterment of your overall health and well-being.

Understanding which exercises might be limited by certain health conditions can help you avoid unnecessary harm and concentrate on safe and beneficial activities. Additionally, being aware of how specific diseases influence your exercise capacities and precautions enables a tailored fitness approach.

Lastly, ensuring that your preventive screenings and tests are current equips you with the confidence to engage in physical activity, knowing that any underlying health issues are effectively managed. These discussions and considerations are equally important for both genders. Despite men and women facing similar risks due to inactivity, like heart disease, diabetes, and osteoporosis, specific factors like menopause-related changes in women warrant additional attention.

Exercising in the golden years isn't solely about maintaining heart health. It's integral to independence, mood enhancement, and boosting the overall quality of life. With the right guidance and personalized approach, older adults can weave a fitness routine into their lifestyle that truly adds life to their years and years to their life.

OVERCOMING YOUR FEARS

Beginning an exercise routine or reintroducing physical activity into your life can be a daunting endeavor, particularly when you're grappling with uncertainties and fears. It's normal to have apprehensions, but it's crucial not to let these fears stop you from embracing a healthier lifestyle. Let's confront these seven common fitness fears and explore how to conquer them:

1. The Fear of Beginning after a Long Hiatus

If it's been a long while since you last engaged in regular exercise, the idea of starting might feel overwhelming. To conquer this fear, start small and gradually build up. Choose low-impact activities like walking or swimming that are easy on your joints and don't require special skills. It's important to remember that every journey begins with a single step, and it's perfectly okay to start slow and progress at your own pace.

2. The Fear of Lifting Weights

Weightlifting can be intimidating, especially if you're new to it or concerned about the risk of injury. But strength training is crucial for maintaining muscle mass and bone density, especially as we age. Start with light weights or resistance bands and gradually increase the resistance as your strength improves. Consider hiring a personal trainer or joining a group class for beginners to learn proper techniques.

3. The Fear of Falling

The fear of falling and injuring oneself is valid, particularly for older adults. Balance exercises and strength training can help reduce this fear by improving your stability and coordination. Tai chi and yoga are excellent choices for enhancing balance. Use supportive equipment like handrails or exercise machines to maintain stability if needed.

4. The Fear of Inducing a Heart Attack

While it's true that physical exertion can stress the heart, the right kind and amount of exercise are beneficial for cardiovascular health. Start with moderate activities and increase your intensity gradually. Ensure that you're cleared by your doctor before starting an exercise regimen, especially if you have a history of heart disease.

5. The Fear of Exacerbating Joint Pain

It's a common misconception that exercise will make joint pain worse. In reality, regular, low-impact activities can help alleviate joint pain by strengthening the muscles around the joints and enhancing flexibility. Consider exercises like swimming, biking, or water aerobics, which are gentle on the knees.

6. The Fear of Disrupting Blood Sugar Control

Physical activity can indeed influence blood sugar levels. However, with proper management, exercise is highly beneficial for people with diabetes. Monitor your blood sugar levels before and after exercise and make the necessary adjustments to your meals or medication with your doctor's guidance.

7. The Fear of Being Too Weak, Old, or Disabled

Age or disability should not preclude you from exercising. Everyone, irrespective of age, ability, or health status can benefit from physical activity. Adapt the exercise to your abilities—seated or low-impact exercises can be effective options. Remember to consult with healthcare professionals or physiotherapists who can help design a safe and suitable exercise plan for you.

Ultimately, these fears, while valid, should not impede your journey toward better health. Start slow, seek professional guidance, listen to your body, and gradually push your boundaries. Fitness is not a destination but a way of life, and it's never too late to start living healthily.

6

REST AND RELAXATION

While it is commonplace to hear about the importance of diet and exercise in controlling blood pressure and safeguarding our heart health, we often overlook two other crucial contributors: quality sleep and effective stress management. Though silent in their operation, these invisible architects of health are powerful in their impact.

The old adage that "Sleep is the best meditation" by the Dalai Lama captures the essence of what this chapter aims to explore. Like a dedicated night-shift worker, quality sleep silently rejuvenates us, repairs our bodies, and prepares us for the battles of the next day. At the same time, effective stress management ensures our emotional armor is ever ready to deal with life's challenges.

In this chapter, we will delve into the intricacies of these critical health components, unraveling their direct and indirect impacts on blood pressure levels. As I uncover the mechanics of restful sleep and the power of keeping stress in check, I'll provide practical, actionable steps that you can incorporate into your daily routines.

Embracing the trifecta of quality sleep, restful breaks, and nurturing tranquility forms a robust defense line in the fight against hypertension. Each component serves as a unique piece of the puzzle that, when combined, boosts your overall heart health. During sleep, our bodies and minds embark on a silent yet essential mission of restoration.

This undisturbed period of rest allows us to mend from the day's wear and tear, leading to a refreshing dawn. However, sleep's elusiveness or insufficiency can set off a chain reaction, increasing stress hormones that may elevate blood pressure and give rise to additional health concerns. Therefore, fostering a sleep environment conducive to restful nights becomes necessary for healthy living.

Interlacing moments of serenity within our day is another key to managing blood pressure. Methods may vary from deep breathing exercises to meditation or simply immersing oneself in a calming hobby. These practices aid in lowering stress levels, effectively serving as an antidote to the constant barrage of life's challenges.

Chronic stress, an often silent but destructive force, is linked to high blood pressure and other health complications. Therefore, like a skilled sailor steering through stormy seas, the ability to keep stress in check becomes an essential skill. Implementing effective stress management techniques aids in sustaining balanced blood pressure levels, contributing to your heart's longevity. By intertwining adequate sleep, moments of calm, and stress management, we build a resilient bulwark for our heart health.

SLEEP

Sleep: It's a universal experience yet cloaked in a veil of mystery. It's a fascinating biological process that scientists are still fervently unraveling. But what is sleep exactly, and why is it so important? Let's dive into this nocturnal world that holds the key to our health and well-being.

Sleep is a natural, recurring state of mind and body characterized by altered consciousness, relatively inhibited sensory activity, reduced interactions with surroundings, and a complex ballet of brain activities. This state is divided into two overarching categories: Rapid Eye Movement (REM) sleep and Non-REM sleep.

Non-REM sleep is further classified into three stages. The first stage represents the bridge from wakefulness to sleep, a period of light sleep when our heartbeat, breathing, and eye movements slow down. The second stage sees the continued slowing of these physiological processes along with brain waves, with occasional bursts of electrical activity. The third stage, often called deep sleep, is vital for feeling refreshed and revitalized the next day.

REM sleep, occurring approximately 90 minutes after falling asleep, is marked by rapid eye movements, increased respiration rate, and brain activity. It's during this stage that vivid dreaming often occurs. These sleep stages form a cycle that repeats multiple times during the night, each stage playing a unique role in the physical and mental rejuvenation process.

The importance of sleep cannot be overstated. It's during this precious time that the body embarks on essential maintenance work. Tissues are repaired, muscles are rebuilt, and hormones are regulated. It's also during sleep that the brain processes and consolidates memories, flushes out toxins, and recharges for the coming day.

The mechanisms of sleep involve an intricate dance between various regions of the brain, hormones, and neurotransmitters. The hypothalamus, a small region at the base of the brain, houses clusters of nerve cells that act as control centers affecting sleep and arousal. Interactions between these nerve cells, hormones such as melatonin, and neurotransmitters like GABA and glycine, all contribute to the timing, quality, and depth of our sleep.

In summary, sleep is an essential biological function with complex stages and mechanisms. It plays a pivotal role in maintaining physical health, cognitive function, and emotional well-being. Understanding the significance of sleep, its stages, and its mechanisms can provide insight into how we can better prioritize and optimize this vital component of our lives.

Sleep and heart health share an intricate and profound relationship that underscores the vital importance of obtaining quality rest. Indeed, when we surrender ourselves to the night, we don't merely drift into a realm of dreams; we also step into a crucial phase of cardiovascular restoration and repair.

Sleep provides a unique window for our heart to ease its ceaseless work. During quality sleep, our heart rate and blood pressure significantly drop, giving our cardiovascular system a much-needed break. This restorative period also offers the opportunity for the heart and vascular system to repair any damage caused by the day's stressors.

Additionally, healthy sleep patterns can promote improved cholesterol levels and reduce inflammation, both of which are paramount in maintaining heart health and minimizing the risk of cardiovascular diseases.

On the flip side, poor sleep or sleep disorders like sleep apnea can have deleterious effects on heart function. These issues can lead to irregular heartbeat, higher blood pressure, increased inflammation, and elevated stress hormones. Such effects do not only put a strain on the heart but can also increase the risk of heart diseases like hypertension, stroke, and heart failure.

In essence, a good night's sleep is not just a luxury—it's a necessity for a healthy heart and a healthier life.

Sleep problems and heart diseases

Sleep isn't merely a passive, restorative state—it's an intricate physiological process that, when disrupted, can have far-reaching implications for cardiovascular health. Various sleep disorders and irregularities have been associated with an increased risk of heart disease, and this connection becomes even more significant as we age.

Sleep apnea, characterized by episodes of halted breathing during sleep, is a common disorder that disrupts the quality of sleep. This condition can cause sudden drops in blood oxygen levels, leading to increased blood pressure and strain on the cardiovascular system, raising the risk of heart disease and stroke.

Moreover, insomnia, a condition where individuals struggle to fall or stay asleep, can lead to chronic sleep deprivation. This lack of sleep may raise stress hormones, increase blood pressure, and stimulate inflammation, creating a conducive environment for heart disease.

As we age, changes in our sleep architecture become evident. Older individuals often experience a reduction in deep

(REM) sleep, encounter more frequent awakenings, and may find it harder to fall asleep. Several factors contribute to these shifts, including changes in circadian rhythm, lifestyle alterations, and health conditions often associated with aging.

Changes in circadian rhythms, our internal biological clock regulating sleep-wake cycles, can lead to earlier sleep and wake times. Lifestyle alterations, such as retirement, can disrupt previous sleep schedules. Moreover, health issues like chronic pain, prostate enlargement, or menopausal symptoms can lead to frequent nighttime awakenings.

These age-related sleep disruptions can further exacerbate the risks of sleep disorders, which can, in turn, negatively impact heart health. Given these complexities, understanding and addressing sleep issues becomes even more critical as we age, not only for heart health but for overall well-being.

As we age, our susceptibility to certain sleep irregularities, which can negatively impact the quality of our slumber and brain oxygen levels, increases. One such notable condition is sleep apnea, marked by distinctive symptoms such as pronounced snoring, intermittent pauses in breathing while asleep, and a pervasive sense of fatigue during the day.

These symptoms don't just disrupt a peaceful night's sleep but also have far-reaching consequences for overall health. One significant aspect relates to the drop in oxygen levels in the brain that occurs during the pauses in breathing, which can result in a host of neurological and cognitive issues.

Furthermore, the disturbances caused by sleep apnea can trigger a cascade of physiological responses. Each episode of halted breathing jolts the body from deep sleep to a lighter stage or even full wakefulness, preventing restorative sleep stages that are key for cognitive functions and physical recovery.

Sleep apnea has also been recognized as a major contributor to hypertension, a topic addressed in an earlier chapter. The repeated oxygen deprivation and subsequent recovery periods lead to increased heart rate and a spike in blood pressure levels, exerting undue stress on the cardiovascular system. Over time, this chronic stress can result in sustained high blood pressure, even during waking hours, amplifying the risk of heart-related complications.

Importantly, the link between sleep apnea and high blood pressure remains robust regardless of other potential contributing factors. Hence, as we grow older, understanding and managing conditions like sleep apnea becomes critical in the pursuit of maintaining not only restful sleep but also long-term cardiovascular health.

Tips for improving sleep

1. **Embrace the Daylight**: Harness the power of natural light during daytime hours. Bright light exposure helps maintain your body's circadian rhythm, the natural internal process that regulates your sleep-wake cycle.
2. **Evening Blue Light Curfew**: Limit your exposure to blue light—emitted by digital screens and artificial lighting—in the evening. This type of light can interfere with your circadian rhythm and the production of melatonin, a hormone that signals your body when it's time to sleep.
3. **Caffeine Curfew**: Avoid consuming caffeinated beverages later in the day. Caffeine can stay elevated in your blood for 6–8 hours, potentially disrupting your sleep if consumed late.
4. **Nap Mindfully**: While daytime naps can be refreshing, long or irregular napping can negatively impact your nighttime sleep quality. If you must nap, keep it short and consistent.
5. **Consistency Is Key**: Try to maintain a regular sleep schedule, going to bed and waking up at the same time each day. This habit can enhance sleep quality by aligning your sleep routine with your body's internal clock.

6. **Alcohol Abstention**: Alcohol can interfere with your sleep cycle and the quality of your sleep, making you more likely to wake up during the night.
7. **Create a Sleep Haven**: Your bedroom environment significantly impacts your ability to fall asleep. Factors such as noise, light, and furniture arrangement should be optimized for sleep.
8. **Cool It Down**: Experiment with different temperatures to find the setting that suits you best. Most people sleep best in a cooler room.
9. **Dinner Timing**: Avoid heavy meals late in the evening. Your body needs time to digest before sleep, and a full stomach can keep you awake.
10. **Evening Relaxation**: Incorporate calming activities into your evening routine. Techniques like meditation, deep breathing, or gentle yoga can help relax your mind and prepare your body for sleep.
11. **The Power of Warmth**: Consider a relaxing bath or shower before bed. The rise and subsequent fall in body temperature can promote feelings of drowsiness.
12. **Assess Your Sleep Health**: If you consistently have difficulty sleeping, you may have a sleep disorder. Consult a healthcare professional for a proper evaluation.
13. **Invest in Comfort**: Your bed, mattress, and pillow play a significant role in sleep quality. Prioritize

comfort and proper support to ensure the best sleep possible.

14. **Move Your Body**: Regular physical activity can help you sleep better. However, try to avoid strenuous workouts close to bedtime as they can interfere with sleep.
15. **Liquid Limitation**: Drinking liquids before bed can lead to disruptive middle-of-the-night trips to the bathroom. Try to minimize your intake in the hours leading up to bedtime.

STRESS MANAGEMENT

Stress is a universal human experience, a psychological and physiological response to life's demands, challenges, and pressures. It's your body's way of protecting you and responding to any kind of demand or threat, essentially a 'fight or flight' response to perceived danger. However, when this response is chronically activated, it can have detrimental effects on your health, including on your heart and blood pressure.

Stress hormones like adrenaline and cortisol are released into your bloodstream when you encounter a stressful situation. These hormones cause an increase in heart rate, a surge in energy, and a narrowing of the blood vessels—all mechanisms designed for survival during a perceived threat.

Unfortunately, repeated or chronic stress can keep these physiological changes activated, leading to persistently high blood pressure, also known as hypertension. Hypertension is a significant risk factor for heart disease and stroke, among other complications.

So, how can we manage stress to control blood pressure better? The answer lies in a combination of lifestyle modifications, relaxation techniques, and healthy coping strategies. Here are a few practical steps:

1. **Mind-Body Practices**: Techniques like meditation, yoga, and deep-breathing exercises can help reduce stress by calming the mind and relaxing the body. Regular practice can help lower the heart rate and blood pressure, promoting overall heart health.
2. **Physical Activity**: Regular exercise releases endorphins, the body's natural mood lifters. It also helps to lower blood pressure by making your heart stronger and more efficient at pumping blood.
3. **Balanced Diet**: Consuming a balanced diet rich in fruits, vegetables, lean protein, and whole grains can keep your body nourished and equipped to handle stress.
4. **Restful Sleep**: Quality sleep is crucial for stress management. Sleep helps your brain function properly and regulate mood, improving your ability to cope with stress.

5. **Positive Social Interactions**: Engaging in social activities, spending time with loved ones, or interacting with a supportive community can provide emotional relief and decrease feelings of stress.
6. **Professional Help**: If stress continues to be overwhelming, consider seeking help from a professional. Therapists or counselors trained in stress management can provide tools and techniques tailored to your unique situation.
7. **Relaxation Techniques**: Progressive muscle relaxation, guided imagery, and biofeedback are techniques that can help you control your body's response to stress, helping to lower blood pressure.
8. **Time Management**: Managing your time effectively can help reduce feelings of pressure and overwhelm, thereby mitigating stress.
9. **Positive Mindset**: Maintaining a positive outlook, practicing gratitude, and employing mindfulness can help counter the negative mental and physical effects of stress.

Stress is an inescapable part of life, but its impact on your health is largely within your control. By identifying stress triggers and developing healthy coping strategies, you can manage stress effectively, promote healthier blood pressure levels, and foster overall well-being. Remember, everyone is different, and it's crucial to find a stress management approach that works for you.

Techniques to reduce stress

Understanding and implementing stress reduction techniques is an essential step toward better overall health. These strategies can help mitigate the effects of stress, particularly its impact on blood pressure levels. Let's explore six such techniques:

1. Breathing Techniques

Deep, focused breathing exercises are quick and effective stress relievers. They work by activating your body's natural relaxation response, slowing your heart rate, and lowering your blood pressure. Simply inhaling deeply through your nose, holding your breath for a few seconds, and then exhaling slowly through your mouth can have a calming effect.

2. Physical Exercise

Regular physical activity is a powerful stress reducer. It promotes the release of endorphins, your body's natural mood boosters. Moreover, it also helps lower blood pressure by improving heart health and enhancing circulation. Choose an exercise routine that you enjoy, whether it's walking, swimming, dancing, or cycling, and try to incorporate it into your daily schedule.

3. Mindfulness

This is the practice of staying fully present in the moment, observing your thoughts and feelings without judgment. Mindfulness can be cultivated through various activities like meditation, mindful eating, or even simple mindful breathing. Practicing mindfulness can help decrease stress by fostering a greater sense of calm and awareness.

4. Progressive Muscle Relaxation

This involves gradually tensing and then relaxing each muscle group in your body, starting from your toes, and working your way up to your head. It's an effective technique for reducing physical tension and mental stress, helping you to feel more relaxed and in control.

5. Visualization

Also known as guided imagery, visualization involves forming peaceful and positive mental images to replace negative or stressful thoughts. Envisioning a tranquil place or scenario can help soothe your mind and body, reducing stress and promoting relaxation.

6. Yoga

Combining physical postures, breathing exercises, and meditation, yoga is an excellent practice for stress management. Regular yoga practice can improve your body's physical response to stress, promoting lower blood pressure, enhanced relaxation, and mental tranquility.

These techniques not only help in mitigating stress but also contribute to the overall sense of well-being. Integrating them into your lifestyle can lead to better blood pressure control, improved emotional health, and enhanced resilience to life's challenges. Remember, consistency is key; make these practices a part of your regular routine to reap their full benefits.

Ways to reduce stress with therapy

Therapeutic methods of stress reduction can add an enjoyable and creative dimension to your stress management regimen. Incorporating these therapies into your lifestyle can offer a holistic approach to maintaining balanced blood pressure levels. Let's explore four such therapies:

1. Aromatherapy

Utilizing aromatic essential oils, aromatherapy can create a calming environment and stimulate the senses, providing relief from stress. Certain scents like lavender, bergamot, or ylang-ylang have been found particularly effective in promoting relaxation. Whether used in diffusers, body oils, or during a bath, the fragrance of these oils can soothe your mind and foster tranquility.

2. Art Therapy

This form of therapy uses the creative process of making art to improve mental well-being. Artistic expression, be it painting, drawing, sculpting, or any other medium, can be a powerful outlet for stress and can help you channel emotions constructively. It doesn't require you to be an artist; the focus is on the process, not the final product.

3. Massage Therapy

A well-executed massage can work wonders in alleviating physical tension and promoting relaxation. By manipulating the body's soft tissues, massage can improve circulation, ease muscle tension, and enhance feelings of overall well-being, thereby helping to mitigate stress-induced blood pressure spikes.

4. Music Therapy

Music has a profound impact on our emotions and can be a potent tool for stress management. Whether you're playing an instrument, singing, or just listening to soothing tunes, music therapy can lower stress levels, reduce heart rate, and create a serene mindset. Choose the type of music that resonates with you, as personal preference plays a significant role in the effectiveness of music therapy.

Exploring these therapeutic avenues to alleviate stress can be rewarding and enjoyable. They provide a multifaceted approach to stress management, helping you find your unique path toward calmness and equanimity, thereby supporting healthier blood pressure levels. Remember, it's not just about reducing stress; it's about enhancing your quality of life and finding joy in the journey.

As we've underscored throughout, securing restful sleep, and effectively navigating stress are key to sustaining optimal blood pressure levels. That said, other lifestyle habits like smoking and alcohol intake can significantly influence your blood pressure.

Consequently, the next chapter will delve deeper into how these behaviors impact blood pressure. We'll also take a look at some useful advice on mitigating or completely ceasing these habits for the sake of enhancing your cardiovascular well-being.

7

KICKING BAD HABITS

"*Most people don't have that willingness to break bad habits. They have a lot of excuses, and they talk like victims.*"

— CARLOS SANTANA

There exist two lifestyle habits that often lurk in the shadow of health discussions—smoking and alcohol consumption. These behaviors can significantly impact blood pressure levels, often escalating them into unhealthy ranges.

In this chapter, I intend to illuminate the intricate links between these habits and heart health, along with a detailed look at the potential effects of these habits on blood pressure. My focus will be on helping you understand these connections and offering practical, actionable, guidance to curtail or completely stop these habits, setting the stage for an improved cardiovascular health landscape.

As Carlos Santana aptly pointed out, breaking free from detrimental habits is often a daunting challenge. People tend to cradle their vices, swaddling them in layers of reasons and perceived helplessness.

Yet, the true essence of self-improvement resides in the courage to acknowledge our weaknesses and the determination to transform them. The path of transformation, however, isn't devoid of hardships. We can easily fall prey to the soothing whispers of excuses, rendering us mere victims in our own narratives. Yet, we must remember that no improvement was ever won by comfort alone. The change that begets improvement is often uncomfortable, sometimes painful, but always worthwhile.

Take smoking and excessive alcohol consumption, for example. They are often clung onto as coping mechanisms, means of socialization, or simply out of habitual routine. However, they wield a double-edged sword, offering momentary relief or pleasure at the expense of long-term health—specifically cardiovascular health.

Asserting control over one's health is a fundamental duty incumbent upon each of us. Instead of merely leaning on the guidance of healthcare practitioners to regulate your well-being, it is vital to initiate an active stance toward self-care. Shaking off detrimental behaviors such as smoking and excessive indulgence in alcohol is an exercise in self-responsibility and self-regulation.

Acknowledging the profound influence these habits can exert on our health and wellness is a critical aspect of managing elevated blood pressure and circumventing associated health complications. Overcoming these ingrained habits can indeed be a Herculean task, but the active pursuit of curbing or discontinuing smoking, along with curtailing alcohol consumption, is nonnegotiable. This implies being answerable for our choices and understanding the significant impact our habits imprint on our comprehensive health status.

SMOKING CESSATION

Smoking cessation is a crucial step toward a healthier life, and its positive impact on blood pressure cannot be overstated. The question that often arises is: "How does smoking elevate blood pressure?" The nicotine in cigarettes stimulates the body to produce adrenaline, which in turn increases heart rate and narrows blood vessels. The result is a temporary spike in blood pressure every time a person smokes.

In the long term, smoking can damage blood vessels, reducing their elasticity and making them more prone to accumulate fatty deposits leading to atherosclerosis—a major risk factor for high blood pressure. Deciding to quit smoking brings immediate and long-term benefits for blood pressure management and overall heart health.

Within 20 minutes of stubbing out the last cigarette, the heart rate and blood pressure begin to normalize. Over the subsequent hours and days, carbon monoxide levels in the blood drop, and oxygen levels rise, improving blood circulation and reducing the strain on the heart.

Several weeks after quitting, the risk of heart attack starts to decline. After about a year, the excess risk of coronary heart disease is half that of a smoker. Over the course of 5 to 15 years, the risk of stroke also reduces to that of a nonsmoker.

Furthermore, quitting smoking can lead to an improvement in blood pressure, often within a few days. This is primarily due to the elimination of the immediate effects of nicotine on blood pressure and heart rate. The extent to which blood pressure drops after quitting smoking can vary depending on individual health circumstances and lifestyle factors, but even a small decrease can have a significant impact on cardiovascular health.

It's important to note, however, that while quitting smoking can lead to an immediate reduction in blood pressure, it does not reverse any damage that has already been done to the blood vessels. Therefore, individuals who have smoked for many years, or who have other risk factors for high blood pressure, should continue to monitor their blood pressure regularly and take steps to maintain a heart-healthy lifestyle.

In essence, cessation of smoking is one of the most impactful actions one can take for one's heart health, and while the journey may be challenging, the rewards are immeasurable. With the right support and commitment, quitting smoking can be a significant stride toward a healthier life, characterized by better blood pressure control and a lower risk of heart disease.

Steps to quit smoking

Embracing the journey to quit smoking involves setting clear goals, planning meticulously, and executing your plan with determination. Here are nine thoughtful steps to guide you through this process:

1. **Establish Your "Quit Day" and Commit**: Begin by setting a specific date as your "Quit Day." This day signifies your commitment to a smoke-free life. As part of this commitment, take a No Smoking pledge —a powerful, personal affirmation of your resolve to quit smoking.
2. **Decide Your Quitting Strategy**: There are different strategies to quit smoking, and you need to choose one that aligns with your habits and preferences. You could quit cold turkey, which means abruptly stopping without any aids, or you could gradually

reduce your smoking frequency until you stop entirely. Alternatively, you could choose to smoke only a part of each cigarette, gradually reducing the amount until you quit completely.

3. **Consult a Healthcare Professional**: Schedule an appointment with your doctor or a healthcare provider. They can provide useful advice and might recommend medicines or support programs that can increase your chances of quitting successfully.

4. **Craft Your Quitting Plan**: Prior to your Quit Day, make a detailed plan that outlines your strategy. This could include tactics to handle cravings, cues to remind you why you're quitting, and rewards for reaching milestones.

5. **Stock Up on Healthy Snacks**: Combat nicotine cravings with healthy snacks. Foods like fruits, nuts, and yogurt can not only help distract you from smoking but also contribute to a healthier lifestyle.

6. **Discover Engaging Distractions**: Identify enjoyable activities to keep you occupied during the times you're usually tempted to smoke. These could include hobbies, exercise, reading, or even puzzles.

7. **Purge Smoking Triggers**: Eliminate any reminder of smoking from your environment. Discard all cigarettes, matches, lighters, ashtrays, and any other tobacco products from your home, office, and car. A clean environment can support your clean break from smoking.

8. **Quit Tobacco on Your Quit Day**: When the day arrives, commit wholeheartedly to your decision. Stick to your plan, lean on your support systems, and remember why you chose to quit.

ALCOHOL CONSUMPTION

While occasional indulgence in a glass of wine, beer, or a favorite cocktail can be part of a balanced lifestyle, it's imperative to remain mindful of the quantity consumed to maintain optimal health. Excessive alcohol intake can lead to detrimental health effects, including the disruption of your cardiovascular system, particularly your blood pressure.

Alcohol has the ability to temporarily increase blood pressure levels, and when consumed in excess over a prolonged period, it can lead to sustained hypertension. The reason lies in the nature of alcohol itself: it is a vasodilator, which means it causes blood vessels to relax and widen. While this might initially seem like it would lower blood pressure, the body counteracts this effect by constricting the blood vessels, leading to an increase in blood pressure.

The recommended daily alcohol intake varies between genders due to physiological differences. For men, it's suggested to limit alcohol consumption to one to two standard drinks per day, whereas, for women, it's advised to stick to one standard drink per day. A standard drink, as defined in the U.S., typically contains about 14 grams of pure alcohol, which equates to 5 ounces of wine, 12 ounces of beer, or 1.5 ounces of distilled spirits.

Remember, these guidelines are averages, not hard-and-fast rules, and individual tolerance and health impact can vary. It's always crucial to listen to your body and consult with healthcare professionals if you're unsure about your alcohol consumption. Balancing enjoyment with moderation is key to maintaining a healthy lifestyle and ensuring that your heart health isn't compromised by overindulgence.

Beers tend to have a lower alcohol concentration than wines, which in turn are generally less potent than distilled spirits. Therefore, the impact on blood pressure can vary depending on the type of drink consumed, and one must consider this when determining what constitutes 'moderate' drinking.

Alcohol can have a direct influence on blood pressure. At intoxicating levels, it will cause vasodilation but at higher levels; it will trigger the release of certain hormones that constrict blood vessels. This will lead to an immediate increase in blood pressure. While this effect is temporary in moderate drinkers, in heavy drinkers, this can result in a sustained elevation of blood pressure, leading to hypertension.

There are specific groups of individuals for whom even moderate alcohol consumption can be harmful. For instance, people diagnosed with certain heart conditions, such as heart rhythm abnormalities or heart failure, should refrain from alcohol intake.

Alcohol can interfere with the normal functioning of the heart and exacerbate these conditions. For instance, in the case of heart rhythm abnormalities, alcohol can trigger episodes of arrhythmia, particularly atrial fibrillation, a condition characterized by an irregular and often rapid heart rate. In the case of heart failure, alcohol can further weaken the heart muscle, impairing its ability to pump blood efficiently.

While the occasional drink may not be harmful to most individuals, it's crucial to understand the potential risks associated with alcohol consumption, especially for those with underlying health conditions.

Consultation with a healthcare professional is highly recommended to determine individual risk factors and set guidelines for safe drinking habits. Maintaining moderation and being mindful of your alcohol intake is a significant step toward preserving cardiovascular health and maintaining healthy blood pressure levels.

Tips on reducing alcohol consumption

Walking on the journey to reduce or eliminate alcohol consumption is a significant commitment to your health. Here are some practical steps to help you along the way:

1. **Put It in Writing**: The first step toward change is often the articulation of your intention. Write down your goal to reduce or stop alcohol consumption. Writing it down gives it a tangible form and serves as a constant reminder of your commitment.
2. **Set a Drinking Goal**: Define what moderation means for you. Decide on the number of days in a week you want to be alcohol-free and the maximum number of drinks you'll have on the days you do consume alcohol.
3. **Keep a Diary of Your Drinking**: Monitoring your consumption can help you recognize patterns and identify triggers. It can provide insights into when and why you drink, which can inform your strategies for reducing consumption.
4. **Empty Your House**: To avoid unnecessary temptation, don't keep alcohol in your home. This ensures that it's not easily accessible, which can significantly help in the initial stages of reducing consumption.

5. **Drink Slowly**: When you do drink, savor it. Take small sips and make a single drink last. This can help reduce the overall quantity consumed.
6. **Choose Alcohol-Free Days**: Dedicate specific days each week when you will abstain from drinking altogether. This helps you break habitual drinking patterns.
7. **Watch for Peer Pressure**: Be mindful of social situations where you might feel pressured to drink. Have a plan to politely decline or opt for nonalcoholic beverages instead.
8. **Keep Busy:** Engage in activities that you enjoy, and that keep you occupied, reducing the likelihood of reaching for a drink out of boredom or habit.
9. **Ask for Support**: Share your goal with trusted friends and family. Their understanding and encouragement can provide a crucial support system as you navigate this journey.
10. **Guard Against Temptation**: Avoid situations where you might be tempted to drink excessively. This could mean opting for social activities that don't revolve around alcohol.
11. **Be Persistent**: Remember, progress is rarely a straight line. There may be setbacks, but don't let them deter you. Persistence is key to achieving your goal.

Reducing or eliminating alcohol consumption is a personal journey and may require tailored strategies based on individual circumstances. Remember, it's okay to seek professional help if you're finding it difficult to manage on your own. Health professionals can provide the necessary support and resources to ensure your success.

As we reach the conclusion of this chapter, we have unraveled the profound influences that smoking and alcohol consumption exert on blood pressure levels. Now, as we turn the page, we're about to delve into another fascinating dimension of heart health—the realm of complementary and alternative interventions.

These strategies can provide additional support in our pursuit of optimal heart health, enhancing your understanding and widening the array of tools we have at our disposal. Stay tuned as we explore this further in the upcoming chapter.

8

BEYOND MEDICATIONS

In this chapter, we embark on a journey to explore the diverse world of complementary and alternative interventions designed to manage blood pressure levels. Just like supporting actors in a play who, though not in the limelight, significantly contribute to the play's success, dietary supplements can offer supportive roles in the pursuit of heart health. They may not be the primary characters in the narrative of managing high blood pressure, yet they contribute substantially to the broader ensemble cast promoting cardiovascular well-being.

Supplements often serve as an adjunct to conventional therapies, adding an extra layer of support. They can provide essential nutrients and substances that our bodies need, supplementing our diet and enhancing our body's natural ability to maintain healthy blood pressure levels.

Keep in mind that supplements are not meant to replace prescribed medication or a healthy lifestyle, but rather complement these primary approaches. This is important because addressing high blood pressure often demands a multi-faceted approach. One that encompasses modifications in lifestyle, the use of prescribed medicines, and other interventions aimed at efficiently reducing blood pressure.

While complementary therapies might not be the frontline defense against high blood pressure, their potential to bolster and synergize with conventional treatments is substantial. Navigating the landscape of high blood pressure management involves harnessing the power of tired-and-tested medical treatments while also leveraging the benefits of supplementary approaches.

Though not a cure in their own right, these complementary measures act as vital pieces in a health puzzle, working in synergy with conventional treatments to create a well-rounded, personalized health plan. Various complementary therapies offer unique advantages, but they all share a common objective: to cultivate an environment that fosters optimal heart health. They provide added value through stress alleviation, nutritional enhancement, and overall wellness improvement.

The goal isn't to upend traditional medical advice or replace prescribed treatments but rather to bolster them. In doing so, we aim to create a more balanced and effective route toward improved heart health.

Moreover, everyone's health journey is distinct, with the ideal blend of treatments being influenced by individual health conditions, personal situations, and preferences. Keeping this in mind, we'll delve into an array of complementary and alternative methods that you might consider integrating into your blood pressure management regimen.

As we delve deeper into this chapter, we'll explore various dietary supplements, their roles, and the evidence backing their efficacy in supporting heart health. Let us journey together into this promising aspect of holistic health management, broadening our understanding of how these supportive actors can help us achieve a healthy and harmonious lifestyle.

OVERVIEW OF COMPLEMENTARY AND ALTERNATIVE THERAPIES

While the phrases "complementary medicine" and "alternative medicine" are frequently used interchangeably and are both encapsulated in the acronym CAM, signifying Complementary and Alternative Medicine, they have distinct meanings. Each term pertains to practices such as herbal treatments or acupuncture, which lie outside conventional Western medicine. However, they differ in how they're utilized.

Complementary medicine refers to the scenario where unconventional therapies are used in conjunction with, or as a complement to, standard Western medicine. The aim is to enhance the effects of traditional treatments, not to replace them.

For instance, meditation, yoga, or acupuncture may be used alongside prescribed medications and a healthy lifestyle to manage blood pressure. The purpose of these complementary methods is to supplement traditional methods, thereby enhancing their effectiveness and offering additional health benefits. They serve as tools that can boost overall well-being, improve stress management, and aid in lifestyle adjustments necessary for controlling blood pressure.

On the other hand, alternative medicine is employed in lieu of traditional medical practices. Instead of utilizing conventional treatments, individuals might opt for these alternative approaches as their primary healthcare strategy. It's essential to understand this distinction to accurately navigate and discuss these healthcare options.

According to Miller (2021), "CAM is frequently seen as bad science but good medicine," illuminates the contrasting views surrounding Complementary and Alternative Medicine. This dichotomy points to the reality that even though these treatments may not always meet the rigorous scientific scrutiny customary in conventional medicine, they often offer valuable benefits to personal health and wellness.

From the lens of rigorous scientific study, CAM therapies are often viewed with a degree of uncertainty. This doubt primarily arises because these practices haven't always undergone the rigorous, large-scale, and double-blind trials that are the gold standard in conventional medical research. Thus, the label "bad science" may be attributed to the perceived deficiency of rigorous scientific evidence supporting these therapies.

However, from the perspective of holistic and patient-focused healthcare, CAM practices are frequently recognized as "good medicine." These therapies aim to enhance health holistically, focusing on the entire individual rather than just the disease. They address various aspects of health, including lifestyle, mental and emotional well-being, and other components contributing to total health. Despite the absence of robust scientific validation, many people have experienced health improvements and an enhanced sense of well-being through these practices.

Thus, while it's essential to scrutinize CAM therapies critically, it's equally crucial to acknowledge their potential merits within a comprehensive approach to healthcare. It's always recommended to consult with a healthcare professional before incorporating any CAM therapies to ensure they align with individual health needs and safety requirements.

MIND-BODY THERAPY

Meditation

Meditation is a time-honored practice that is rooted in various traditions across the world. It is a technique focused on bringing tranquility to the mind and the body by concentrating on a single thought, object, or process, such as breathing. This practice has evolved over centuries and today exists in various forms, each with its unique method but sharing the common goal of attaining inner peace and relaxation.

It's intriguing to note how this seemingly simple mind-body practice can impact physical health parameters, specifically blood pressure. Our bodies respond to stress with a surge of hormones, including cortisol and adrenaline, which temporarily increase blood pressure.

This temporary rise in blood pressure is natural and not typically a concern. However, continuous exposure to stress, and hence a persistently elevated level of these hormones, can lead to sustained high blood pressure—a risk factor for heart disease.

Meditation enters the scene as a powerful stress-busting tool that can mitigate this risk. By invoking a state of deep relaxation, meditation encourages the body to lower the production of stress hormones, reducing their impact on the cardiovascular system. This state of tranquility not only tempers the immediate stress response but also contributes to reducing baseline blood pressure levels over time.

Moreover, scientific investigations have uncovered substantial evidence supporting the positive influence of consistent meditation on blood pressure. In particular, transcendental meditation, a specialized variant of the practice, has been linked with appreciable decreases in both upper (systolic) and lower (diastolic) blood pressure readings. It involves the silent repetition of a personal mantra, which is a word or phrase in a specific manner. The objective is to induce a state of relaxed awareness that facilitates the release of stress and fatigue from the mind and body.

In a study conducted by Joanne Kraenzle Schneider, Chuntana Reangsing, and Danny G. Willis (2022), the impact of this particular form of meditation on blood pressure was found. Their findings indicated that TM could lead to a modest decrease in blood pressure, although this effect tends to diminish after approximately three months. Additionally, they observed that older adults above the age of 65 appeared to derive greater benefits compared to younger adults.

However, it is important to note that the researchers were cautious in interpreting these findings. They emphasized that Transcendental Meditation should be viewed as one aspect of a heart-healthy lifestyle rather than a standalone solution for high blood pressure.

This perspective aligns with the broader philosophy of complementary and alternative medicine, which promotes holistic and comprehensive approaches to health and well-being. Therefore, while TM may not produce significant and long-lasting reductions in blood pressure on its own, it can still contribute to an overall strategy for managing blood pressure and promoting heart health, particularly when combined with other lifestyle adjustments such as dietary changes, exercise, and stress management.

Another study conducted by James W. Anderson, Chunxu Liu, and Richard J Kryscio delves deeper into the impact of Transcendental Meditation on blood pressure. The findings suggest that practicing Transcendental Meditation can potentially lead to clinically significant changes, with systolic blood pressure decreasing by approximately 4.7 mm Hg and diastolic blood pressure decreasing by 3.2 mm Hg.

Although these reductions may appear modest, they can hold great clinical importance. Even a slight decrease in blood pressure can substantially reduce the risk of heart disease and stroke. Therefore, these findings highlight the potential value of Transcendental Meditation as part of a comprehensive approach to managing high blood pressure.

In addition to its effects on blood pressure, the researchers also observed a range of other health benefits associated with regular Transcendental Meditation practice. These benefits encompass anxiety reduction, improved sleep quality, and enhanced overall well-being.

Consequently, this study not only reinforces the potential of Transcendental Meditation as a tool for blood pressure management but also emphasizes that the advantages of such practices extend beyond physical health. The promotion of mental and emotional well-being, better sleep, and reduced anxiety are all integral aspects of a holistic approach to health. This further underscores the value of incorporating techniques like Transcendental Meditation into a comprehensive health and wellness strategy.

How to Meditate

Meditation can seem like an intricate and daunting practice, but its core concept is straightforward—stilling the mind to bring about a sense of inner peace and self-awareness. Here's a simplified step-by-step guide to meditation:

1. **Find a Peaceful Location**: Choose a serene spot where you won't be disturbed during your meditation session. It could be a quiet room in your house, a tranquil garden, or even a quiet park.
2. **Choose a Comfortable Position**: Sit comfortably. You can opt to sit on a chair, cross-legged on the floor, or even lie down if that's more comfortable for you. The goal is to find a position where you can remain relaxed yet attentive.
3. **Focus Your Attention**: Close your eyes and start focusing on your breath. Observe the sensation of

your breath as it flows in and out. Try not to control your breath but rather just observe its natural rhythm.

4. **Be Mindful:** Your mind will inevitably wander, and that's okay. Whenever you realize that your thoughts have drifted, gently redirect your focus back to your breath without judging yourself.

5. **Start Small and Gradually Increase Duration**: Start by meditating for just a few minutes a day, then gradually increase your practice time as you feel comfortable. Even a few minutes of meditation can make a difference.

6. **Practice Regularly**: Consistency is key in meditation. Make it a part of your daily routine to get the most benefit out of the practice.

Remember, meditation is not about attaining perfection but rather about improving awareness and acceptance. It's perfectly normal to have days when meditation feels more challenging. What matters most is that you persist and continue the practice.

Also, while meditation is a powerful tool in managing stress and improving blood pressure, it should not be considered a standalone treatment for high blood pressure. It is best utilized as a complementary approach alongside traditional blood pressure management strategies. As always, any changes to your health regimen should be discussed with a healthcare professional.

Yoga

Yoga offers a holistic approach to managing blood pressure by addressing both physical and mental well-being. Through regular practice, yoga has been shown to effectively reduce stress levels, which can contribute to high blood pressure. By engaging in various yoga techniques, individuals can experience a decrease in stress hormones and a promotion of relaxation, ultimately leading to lower blood pressure levels.

In addition to stress reduction, yoga can enhance overall fitness and cardiovascular health. Certain forms of yoga, such as Vinyasa or Power Yoga, involve dynamic movements and increased physical exertion, which can improve cardiovascular endurance. This aspect of yoga is particularly advantageous for individuals with high blood pressure, as it helps to strengthen the heart and improve its efficiency.

A comprehensive study published in Mayo Clinic Proceedings in 2019 further supports the positive effects of yoga on blood pressure. The research focused on overweight, middle-aged adults with high blood pressure who practiced yoga for about an hour five times a week over a period of 13 weeks. The study revealed significant reductions in blood pressure among the participants. Furthermore, when the yoga sessions incorporated specific breathing techniques and meditation, the improvements in blood pressure were even more pronounced.

These findings emphasize the potential of yoga as a valuable tool in blood pressure management. By integrating physical postures, breathing exercises, and meditation, yoga provides a comprehensive approach to promoting cardiovascular health and reducing stress. As with any exercise or therapeutic practice, it's advisable to consult with a healthcare professional before starting a yoga routine, especially for individuals with pre-existing medical conditions.

Yoga Poses – Lower Blood Pressure

Incorporating yoga into your lifestyle can be a powerful tool in managing and reducing high blood pressure. Yoga combines physical postures, controlled breathing, and mindfulness to promote overall health and well-being.

Along with its numerous benefits for the body and mind, yoga has been shown to positively affect blood pressure levels. By practicing specific yoga poses that target relaxation, stress reduction, and circulation you can support your cardiovascular health and work toward maintaining a healthy blood pressure range.

In this section, I will take you through six yoga poses that are particularly beneficial for reducing high blood pressure. By integrating these poses into your regular practice, you can harness the therapeutic benefits of yoga and embark on a journey toward better heart health and overall well-being.

1. Balasana (Child's Pose): Balasana, or Child's Pose, is a gentle and relaxing yoga posture that can help reduce high blood pressure. Start kneeling on the mat with your toes touching and knees slightly apart. Slowly lower your hips toward your heels and rest your forehead on the mat. Extend your arms alongside your body or place them gently on the mat above your head. Take slow, deep breaths, allowing your body to relax and release tension. Balasana promotes a sense of calmness and relaxation, helping to reduce stress and lower blood pressure.

2. Paschimottanasana (Seated Forward Bend): Paschimottanasana, or Seated Forward Bend, is a seated yoga pose that stretches the entire back of the body, promoting relaxation and relieving tension. Sit on the mat with your legs extended in front of you. Slowly bend forward from the hips, reaching your hands toward your feet or resting them on your shins or thighs. Keep your spine long and your gaze forward. Breathe deeply and relax into the pose, allowing your body to gently release tension. Paschimottanasana helps to calm the mind, reduce stress, and regulate blood pressure.

3. Baddha Konasana (Bound Angle Pose): Baddha Konasana, or Bound Angle Pose, is a seated posture that opens the hips and promotes relaxation. Sit on the mat with your legs bent and the soles of your feet touching each other. Hold your feet or ankles with your hands and gently press your knees toward the floor. Sit tall and lengthen your spine, allowing your hips to open and your inner thighs to stretch.

Take slow, deep breaths, focusing on relaxing your body and mind. Baddha Konasana helps relieve anxiety, improve circulation, and support healthy blood pressure.

4. Janu Sirsasana (Head-to-Knee Pose): Janu Sirsasana, or Head-to-Knee Pose, is a seated forward bend that stretches the hamstrings and calms the nervous system. Sit on the mat with one leg extended and the sole of the other foot against your inner thigh. Slowly fold forward, reaching toward your extended leg with your hands. Keep your spine long and breathe deeply as you relax into the pose. Janu Sirsasana helps to release tension, reduce stress, and promote healthy blood pressure levels.

5. Virasana (Hero Pose) with extended exhale breathing: Virasana, or Hero Pose, is a kneeling posture that opens the chest, promotes relaxation, and supports healthy blood pressure. Start by kneeling on the mat with your knees together and your feet slightly apart. Sit back on your heels and lengthen your spine. Place your hands on your thighs or rest them on your knees. Take slow, deep breaths, and as you exhale, extend the length of your breath, allowing your exhalations to be longer than your inhalations. Virasana, with extended exhale breathing, helps to activate the parasympathetic nervous system, reduce stress, and regulate blood pressure.

6. Savasana (Corpse Pose): Savasana, or Corpse Pose, is a deeply relaxing and restorative posture that allows the body and mind to fully relax. Lie on your back with your legs extended and your arms resting alongside your body, palms facing up. Close your eyes and focus on your breath, allowing it to flow naturally and deeply. Release any tension in your body and surrender to a state of complete relaxation. Savasana helps to reduce stress, lower blood pressure, and promote overall well-being. It allows for deep rest and rejuvenation, supporting the body's natural healing processes.

VITAMINS

Vitamins are essential organic compounds that are required in small amounts for the body's normal functioning. They play a crucial role in various physiological processes, such as metabolism, growth, and maintenance of overall health. Vitamins are classified into two main types: fat-soluble and water-soluble.

Fat-soluble vitamins, as the name suggests, dissolve and are stored in the body's fatty tissues. These include vitamins A, D, E, and K. Fat-soluble vitamins are absorbed through the intestines and dietary fats and stored in the liver and fatty tissues for future use. Because they can be stored, excess consumption of fat-soluble vitamins can potentially lead to toxicity.

On the other hand, water-soluble vitamins, including vitamin C and the B-complex vitamins (such as B1, B2, B3, B5, B6, B7, B9, and B12) are not stored in the body to a significant extent. They dissolve in water and are easily absorbed into the bloodstream. Water-soluble vitamins are not stored in large quantities, and any excess amounts are excreted through urine. Therefore, regular intake of water-soluble vitamins is important to meet the body's requirements.

Both types of vitamins are essential for maintaining optimal health, but it's important to note that the body's requirements for each vitamin may vary. A balanced diet that includes a variety of foods can provide an adequate intake of vitamins. However, in certain cases, such as pregnancy, illness, or specific dietary restrictions, supplementation may be recommended under the guidance of a healthcare professional to ensure sufficient vitamin intake.

MINERALS

Minerals are vital micronutrients that our bodies require in relatively small amounts to support various physiological functions. They are essential for maintaining overall health and well-being. Let's explore some of the different types of minerals and their roles in the body, particularly their importance for individuals with high blood pressure:

1. **Calcium**: Calcium is well known for its role in promoting strong bones and teeth. It also plays a crucial role in regulating blood pressure by assisting in constricting and relaxing blood vessels.

2. **Magnesium:** Magnesium is involved in over 300 biochemical reactions in the body. It helps relax blood vessels, thereby contributing to the maintenance of healthy blood pressure levels.
3. **Potassium:** Potassium is an electrolyte that helps balance the fluids and minerals in the body. It plays a vital role in regulating blood pressure by counteracting the effects of sodium and supporting healthy heart function.
4. **Sodium:** While excessive sodium intake can contribute to high blood pressure, a moderate amount of sodium is necessary for maintaining fluid balance and supporting proper nerve and muscle function.
5. **Zinc:** Zinc is involved in numerous enzymatic reactions and plays a crucial role in immune function, wound healing, and cell division. It indirectly contributes to blood pressure regulation by supporting overall cardiovascular health.
6. **Iron:** Iron is essential for the production of red blood cells, which transport oxygen throughout the body. Adequate iron levels are crucial for maintaining optimal blood pressure and preventing conditions associated with iron deficiency.

For individuals with high blood pressure, maintaining appropriate mineral levels is important. A balanced diet that includes a variety of nutrient-rich foods such as fruits, vegetables, whole grains, lean proteins, and low-fat dairy products can provide an adequate intake of minerals.

In this regard, it is important to remember that certain medical conditions or medications may affect mineral levels, so consulting with a healthcare professional or registered dietitian is recommended to tailor a dietary plan that suits individual needs. By incorporating a variety of mineral-rich foods into their diet, blood pressure patients can support their overall health and contribute to the management of their condition.

FOOD OR SUPPLEMENTS

When it comes to obtaining vitamins and minerals, it is generally recommended to prioritize food as the primary source. Whole foods provide a wide array of essential nutrients, along with other beneficial compounds such as fiber and antioxidants.

The body is designed to absorb and utilize vitamins and minerals more efficiently from food sources, as they come packaged with other synergistic components that work together for optimal absorption and utilization. While supplements can be helpful in certain situations, such as addressing specific deficiencies or supporting certain health conditions, they should not replace a well-balanced diet.

Whole foods offer the added advantage of providing a diverse range of nutrients and phytochemicals that support overall health and well-being. Therefore, focusing on a nutrient-rich diet, including a variety of fruits, vegetables, whole grains, lean proteins, and healthy fats, is the best approach to meet the body's vitamin and mineral needs.

In most cases, the absorption of vitamins and minerals from natural food sources tends to be more efficient compared to their synthetic counterparts in supplement form.

Choosing a well-rounded, nutrient-dense diet over relying solely on supplements provides a multitude of benefits, as whole foods offer a wide spectrum of nutrients, fiber, and antioxidants that contribute to overall health and well-being. However, it's important to acknowledge that relying solely on food for all necessary vitamins and minerals can pose challenges.

Access to a diverse range of nutrient-rich foods may be limited for some individuals due to various factors such as geographical location, economic constraints, or personal dietary restrictions. Additionally, factors like soil quality, food processing, and cooking methods can affect the nutrient content of foods, making it challenging to guarantee sufficient intake through diet alone.

In such cases, supplements can be a helpful tool to fill potential nutritional gaps and address specific deficiencies. They can provide concentrated doses of certain vitamins and minerals, especially when prescribed by healthcare professionals. It is crucial, though, to approach supplements as complementary to a healthy diet rather than a substitute.

Relying solely on supplements while neglecting a balanced eating pattern can lead to a lack of other essential nutrients and the associated benefits they provide. Striking a balance between obtaining nutrients from whole foods and considering targeted supplementation when necessary can help ensure optimal nutrient intake.

DIETARY SUPPLEMENTS

Dietary supplements are products intended to supplement one's diet and provide additional nutrients, such as vitamins, minerals, herbs, or other botanicals, amino acids, or enzymes. They come in various forms, including capsules, tablets, powders, liquids, or even energy bars.

The benefits of dietary supplements lie in their ability to fill potential nutritional gaps and support overall health and well-being. They can be particularly beneficial for individuals with specific dietary restrictions, limited access to nutrient-rich foods, or increased nutrient needs due to certain life stages or health conditions.

Supplements can help bridge nutritional deficiencies and ensure adequate intake of essential vitamins, minerals, and other vital nutrients. It's also important to keep in mind that prior to incorporating any dietary supplements into your routine, it is crucial to consult with your doctor to verify that they will not interfere with any medications you are currently taking or result in any undesirable consequences.

Even though natural supplements may be considered safe, it is essential to recognize that they can still induce side effects, particularly when consumed in excessive quantities or for prolonged durations. Additionally, it is advisable to undergo laboratory tests and undergo a micronutrient assessment to gain insights into your current nutrient levels before initiating any supplement plan.

MICRONUTRIENT TESTS

A micronutrient test is a specialized assessment that offers valuable information regarding the presence of any nutrient deficiencies or imbalances within your body. By analyzing your blood or other bodily samples, this test can identify specific micronutrient levels and provide insights into your individual nutritional needs.

This knowledge can be instrumental in determining which dietary supplements may be most beneficial for addressing any deficiencies or imbalances. To ensure an accurate interpretation of the results and appropriate supplementation, it is recommended to consult with your healthcare provider. They can guide you in selecting the most suitable micronutrient test for your circumstances and help you understand the significance of the findings.

Understanding your micronutrient status through testing allows you and your healthcare provider to develop a more targeted approach to your nutritional supplementation. By identifying the nutrients that may be lacking or imbalanced, you can choose the appropriate dietary supplements to address those specific needs.

It's important to remember that dietary supplements are designed to complement a healthy and balanced diet, not to serve as a substitute for it. Emphasizing whole foods as the primary source of nutrients is essential for overall well-being. Supplements should be used judiciously and, only when necessary, to support and enhance your overall health and wellness journey.

SUPPLEMENTS FOR YOU

Various supplements have a crucial role in meeting the dietary requirements of individuals with hypertension. They serve as a valuable source of extra nutrients that may be deficient in their regular diet, aiding in the promotion of overall well-being and the regulation of blood pressure.

Specific supplements like magnesium, potassium, and CoQ10 have been linked to the reduction of blood pressure levels. Additionally, the inclusion of omega-3 fatty acids from fish oil supplements can contribute to cardiovascular health. These supplements offer an effective means of supplementing one's diet to address nutritional gaps and support the management of blood pressure.

Some of the most important supplements include the following:

Magnesium: Magnesium is crucial for regulating blood pressure and muscle function. Optimal magnesium levels have been linked to lower blood pressure.

Vitamin D: Insufficient vitamin D has been associated with hypertension. Taking vitamin D supplements may help maintain healthy blood pressure.

B vitamins: B vitamins, such as folate, vitamin B6, and vitamin B12, play a role in cardiovascular health and maintaining optimal blood pressure.

Potassium: Essential for balancing sodium levels, potassium helps support healthy blood pressure. Adequate intake through supplements or potassium-rich foods is beneficial.

CoQ10: Coenzyme Q10 (CoQ10) is an antioxidant involved in cellular energy production. Studies suggest that CoQ10 supplementation may contribute to lower blood pressure.

L-arginine: L-arginine, an amino acid, promotes the production of nitric oxide, which aids in blood vessel relaxation and improves blood flow, potentially benefiting blood pressure.

Vitamin C: As an antioxidant, vitamin C may enhance blood vessel function and promote healthy blood pressure levels.

Beetroot: Rich in nitrates, beetroot can be converted to nitric oxide, supporting blood vessel dilation, and potentially reducing blood pressure.

Garlic: Garlic has long been recognized for its cardiovascular benefits, including maintaining healthy blood pressure.

Fish oil: Omega-3 fatty acids in fish oil offer cardiovascular advantages, including support for healthy blood pressure.

Probiotics: Select probiotic strains may contribute to cardiovascular health, including the maintenance of healthy blood pressure levels.

Melatonin: Melatonin, a hormone involved in sleep-wake cycles, may modestly impact blood pressure regulation.

Green tea: Green tea contains catechins, compounds with antioxidants and blood pressure-lowering properties.

Ginger: Ginger has been studied for potential cardiovascular benefits, including its impact on healthy blood pressure levels.

Vitamin K2: Vitamin K2 aids in calcium metabolism and vascular health, potentially influencing blood pressure regulation.

Caution: When contemplating the utilization of vitamins for managing blood pressure, it is crucial to approach it with caution and take necessary precautions. The foremost step is to seek advice from your healthcare professional before initiating any new supplements.

If you are taking blood thinners, avoid the consumption of Vitamin K2. Blood thinners work by inhibiting the formation of blood clotting factors that depend on vitamin K. Taking vitamin K can interfere with the intended effects of blood thinners, counteracting their effectiveness. It is important to consult with your healthcare provider or pharmacist to understand potential interactions and to ensure the safe and appropriate use of Vitamin K2 or any other supplements while on blood thinners.

COMMIT TO THE JOURNEY

If lifestyle modifications alone do not yield the desired results in lowering blood pressure within a span of six months, a recent scientific statement by the American Heart Association proposes maintaining those healthy habits while also contemplating the inclusion of blood pressure-lowering medications.

The journey of managing hypertension can be a lengthy endeavor, but the rewards that come with it are unquestionably worthwhile. Lowering blood pressure requires a holistic approach, encompassing medications, lifestyle modifications, and complementary or alternative therapies.

It's important to recognize that the desired outcomes may not manifest instantly; rather, it may take several weeks or even months to witness the full effects of these interventions. Despite the challenges that may arise during this process, maintaining unwavering commitment and adhering to your personalized plan is fundamental to achieving success.

Perseverance and resilience play vital roles, as consistency is the key to attaining long-lasting results. Even when progress appears gradual, faithfully integrating the recommended changes into your daily routine will contribute to a healthier and more enriching life.

It's crucial to remain mindful of the fact that the path to improved blood pressure management is an ongoing journey that demands patience and unwavering dedication. In the upcoming chapter, we will delve into understanding the consequences of not checking high blood pressure.

9

THE HIDDEN DANGERS

Various risks and complications exist with uncontrolled hypertension. In fact, a fundamental challenge in the field of medicine lies in the realm of uncertainty, which permeates the experiences of patients, doctors, and society at large. In *Complications: A Surgeon's Notes on an Imperfect Science* Atul Gawande remarkably stated that despite the progress we have made in understanding human health, diseases, and their treatments, the pervasive nature of uncertainty remains elusive.

As a patient, navigating through this uncertainty can be emotionally distressing, while doctors face the constant struggle of grappling with the vast expanse of the unknown. It becomes evident that the essence of medical care resides not solely in what is known but rather in acknowledging and addressing what remains uncertain. Uncertainty forms the bedrock of medicine, and the ability to navigate it wisely becomes a defining factor in both the patient's and doctor's journey.

The field of medicine encompasses more than just precise calculations and definitive solutions. Even with the most advanced treatments available, there are inherent uncertainties and unknown factors that permeate the management of health conditions.

However, in the case of high blood pressure, the risks and potential complications associated with uncontrolled hypertension are widely acknowledged and substantial. Despite some degree of uncertainty regarding the ideal treatment approach, the dangers posed by unmanaged high blood pressure are evident.

They range from detrimental effects on vital organs like the heart, brain, and kidneys to an increased susceptibility to life-threatening events such as stroke. By prioritizing blood pressure management and maintaining close collaboration with healthcare professionals, individuals can effectively minimize the risks and uncertainties.

Gaining an understanding of these risks and complications is paramount to taking proactive measures in blood pressure management and ensuring optimal long-term health. Moreover, when it comes to high blood pressure, risks and complications are interconnected concepts, each with its own distinct meaning.

- Risks pertain to factors or conditions that heighten the probability of a particular event occurring.
- Complications, on the other hand, encompass the adverse health outcomes that can arise as a consequence of a given condition.

Furthermore, risks encompass various factors that can increase the likelihood of developing the condition or experiencing related health issues. These factors may include family history, certain lifestyle choices, or underlying medical conditions.

On the other hand, complications associated with high blood pressure involve the negative health consequences that can manifest when the condition is left uncontrolled. These complications can range from cardiovascular problems, such as heart attack or stroke, to damage to organs like the kidneys or brain.

RISKS AND COMPLICATIONS OF UNCONTROLLED HYPERTENSION

When it comes to high blood pressure, several risks and complications can make matters worse. In this section, we'll be walking through some of the major ones.

Damaged and narrowed arteries

Increased blood pressure can result in harm to the inner lining of arteries. This damage can worsen when fats from the diet accumulate in the bloodstream. The combined effect of arterial damage and fat buildup can diminish the flexibility of artery walls, impeding the smooth flow of blood throughout the body. This reduced blood flow over an extended period can give rise to various complications, such as heart disease, stroke, and damage to other organs and tissues in the body.

Aneurysm

Consistently elevated blood pressure increases the pressure on weakened areas of the arteries. This prolonged pressure can cause further weakening of the arterial wall, potentially leading to an aneurysm. As the artery endures heightened stress, the weakened segment may enlarge and possibly rupture, resulting in severe internal bleeding that poses a life-threatening risk.

While not all aneurysms are directly caused by high blood pressure, hypertension can contribute to their formation and elevate the risk of complications. Maintaining blood pressure within a healthy range is crucial to reduce the chances of aneurysm development and rupture.

Through effective blood pressure management involving lifestyle adjustments, prescribed medications, and regular monitoring, individuals can significantly decrease the likelihood of developing an aneurysm. Collaborating closely with healthcare professionals enables the creation of a comprehensive plan encompassing routine blood pressure checks, the adoption of healthy eating habits, regular exercise, stress reduction techniques, and adherence to prescribed medications.

Always remember that preventing aneurysms begins with maintaining a healthy blood pressure level. By taking proactive measures to manage hypertension, you can safeguard those blood vessels and diminish the risks associated with aneurysm formation.

Damage to the heart

Elevated blood pressure disrupts the functioning of the endothelial system, posing a considerable risk for the development of atherosclerotic disease, coronary artery disease, and peripheral arterial disease (Tackling & Borhade, 2022). Hypertension can cause damage to the arteries and result in their narrowing, impeding the flow of blood to the heart.

This reduction in blood flow can manifest as chest pain, irregular heart rhythms, and, in severe cases, heart attacks. When left uncontrolled, high blood pressure can lead to the narrowing and impairment of arteries, depriving the heart of sufficient blood supply.

Enlarged left ventricle

Elevated blood pressure forces the heart to exert more effort in pumping blood across the body. This added strain can result in the thickening of the left ventricle of the heart, heightening the chances of heart attack, heart failure, and sudden cardiac death.

When high blood pressure remains uncontrolled, the left ventricle of the heart may thicken, compromising its ability to function effectively. This condition, referred to as left ventricular hypertrophy, increases the susceptibility to severe heart complications, including heart attacks and heart failure.

Heart failure

As time passes, elevated blood pressure can exert pressure on the heart, leading to strain. This strain can result in the weakening of the heart muscle and a decline in its efficiency. If the strain persists over an extended period, it can eventually lead to heart failure, where the heart's ability to pump blood adequately becomes compromised.

Damage to the brain

Transient Ischemic Attack (TIA)

A transient ischemic attack (TIA) is considered a mild form of stroke. It occurs when there is a temporary blockage or reduction in blood flow to a specific area of the brain, usually caused by a blood clot. Unlike a stroke, the symptoms of a TIA are similar but brief and do not result in lasting damage.

The blockage in a blood vessel supplying the brain can occur due to damage caused by high blood pressure or high cholesterol. Additionally, a blood clot from another location, such as the heart or neck blood vessels, can also travel to the brain and cause a TIA.

Often referred to as a ministroke, a TIA serves as a warning sign that a more severe stroke may occur in the future. It is crucial to address high blood pressure as it can contribute to the formation of hardened arteries or blood clots, increasing the risk of experiencing a TIA.

Stroke

Insufficient oxygen and nutrients reaching the brain can result in a stroke as the cells in the brain start to perish. High blood pressure can be detrimental to blood vessels in the brain, causing them to narrow, rupture, or leak, thereby increasing the likelihood of a stroke.

Furthermore, hypertension raises the risk of blood clots forming within the arteries that supply the brain, obstructing the flow of blood and potentially leading to a stroke. By damaging blood vessels and promoting clot formation, high blood pressure poses a significant threat to the occurrence of a stroke.

Dementia

Vascular dementia, a specific form of dementia, can manifest when the arteries supplying blood to the brain undergo narrowing or blockage. This leads to the restriction of blood flow and causes harm to brain cells.

Additionally, a stroke that disrupts blood flow to the brain can contribute to the development of vascular dementia, as it inflicts considerable damage and loss of brain cells, consequently impairing cognitive abilities and memory. In both cases, the compromised blood flow and subsequent damage to brain cells are key factors in the onset of vascular dementia—highlighting the critical importance of maintaining healthy blood circulation to preserve cognitive function.

Mild Cognitive Impairment

Mild cognitive impairment represents a transitional stage between typical age-related changes in cognition and more severe forms of dementia, characterized by noticeable alterations in memory and comprehension (NHS, 2019).

Emerging evidence indicates that elevated blood pressure may play a role in the onset of mild cognitive impairment.

Research suggests that high blood pressure could be a contributing factor in the development of these cognitive changes, highlighting the potential link between hypertension and the early stages of cognitive decline. Understanding the impact of blood pressure on cognitive health is crucial in identifying strategies to mitigate the risk and promote optimal brain function.

Damage to the kidneys

Kidney scarring (glomerulosclerosis)

High blood pressure can also impact the kidneys. A common condition that can develop is known as "Glomerulosclerosis." In this condition, tiny blood vessels within the kidneys undergo scarring.

As a result, the kidneys lose their ability to efficiently filter waste and fluid from the blood. The progression of glomerulosclerosis can ultimately lead to kidney failure, a critical and potentially life-threatening condition.

When the kidneys fail, they are unable to adequately perform their vital functions of removing waste and excess fluid from the body. Recognizing the implications of glomerulosclerosis is crucial as it highlights the significance of preserving kidney health and seeking appropriate medical intervention to prevent or manage kidney failure.

Kidney failure

High blood pressure stands as a primary contributor to the development of kidney failure. This arises from the potential damage inflicted upon the blood vessels responsible for supplying the kidneys, impeding their proper functioning.

When the kidneys are unable to efficiently filter waste and excess fluid from the blood, the accumulation of harmful levels within the body can ensue, leading to severe complications and, in some cases, kidney failure. To address kidney failure resulting from uncontrolled hypertension, treatment options such as dialysis or kidney transplantation may be necessary.

However, individuals can actively reduce their risk of kidney failure by effectively managing their blood pressure and collaborating with healthcare professionals to prevent and control kidney disease. Taking proactive steps in these regards significantly contributes to preserving kidney health and overall well-being.

Damage to the eyes

Retinopathy refers to the impairment of blood vessels in the retina caused by uncontrolled hypertension. This condition can give rise to various vision issues, including blurred vision and, in severe cases, complete vision loss.

Moreover, the damage inflicted upon the retinal blood vessels can result in bleeding within the eye, which presents a significant and potentially serious complication. Individuals with both high blood pressure and diabetes face an elevated risk of developing retinopathy, as these conditions collectively contribute to the deterioration of blood vessels in the eye. Thus, it is crucial to manage blood pressure levels effectively and address related conditions to minimize the risk of retinopathy and safeguard visual health.

Fluid buildup under the retina (Choroidopathy)

Choroidopathy is a condition that affects the blood vessels in the eye and can have detrimental effects on vision. It can manifest as distorted or blurry vision, and in more severe cases, it may result in scarring that can permanently impair vision.

The damage caused by choroidopathy can lead to various vision problems, including the distortion of images, making it difficult for individuals to see clearly. Consequently, managing choroidopathy is crucial to preserve visual acuity and minimize the impact on daily activities. Regular eye examinations and appropriate treatment can help mitigate the effects of choroidopathy and maintain optimal vision.

Nerve damage (Optic Neuropathy)

Impaired blood flow can adversely affect the optic nerve, leading to vision loss or intraocular bleeding. Blockage of blood flow can result in damage to the optic nerve, causing the accumulation of blood within the eye or even partial or complete loss of vision.

When the optic nerve is compromised due to inadequate blood supply, it hampers the transmission of visual signals to the brain, leading to visual disturbances. It is important to address the obstruction of blood flow promptly to minimize the risk of optic nerve damage and preserve visual function. Seeking medical attention and adopting appropriate interventions can help mitigate the potential consequences of vision.

Sexual Dysfunction

In men aged 50 and above, it is common to encounter erectile dysfunction, a condition characterized by the inability to achieve or sustain an erection. However, men with high blood pressure face an even higher likelihood of experiencing erectile dysfunction, as hypertension can restrict the blood flow to the penis.

Similarly, women with high blood pressure may also encounter challenges in sexual functioning. High blood pressure can lead to diminished blood flow to the vagina, resulting in decreased sexual desire, difficulty getting aroused, vaginal dryness, and difficulties in achieving orgasm. These effects on sexual health emphasize the importance of managing blood pressure to promote a satisfying and fulfilling sexual experience for both men and women.

PREVENTING RISKS AND COMPLICATIONS

To prevent the risks and complications associated with uncontrolled high blood pressure, a comprehensive approach that combines lifestyle modifications and medication is often necessary. Here are some strategies that can help you in dealing with these complications:

- Regularly monitor your blood pressure and collaborate with your healthcare provider to develop a personalized management plan.
- Implement lifestyle changes that support healthy blood pressure levels, such as adopting a heart-healthy diet, engaging in regular physical activity, managing stress effectively, and quitting smoking.
- Adhere to prescribed medications as directed by your doctor and be mindful of any potential side effects or interactions with other medications, supplements, or food.
- Manage other underlying health conditions that can contribute to high blood pressure or increase your

- risk of complications, such as diabetes or high cholesterol.
- Pay attention to any symptoms or warning signs of a complication, such as chest pain, shortness of breath, severe headache, or changes in vision, and seek prompt medical attention if they arise.
- By taking a proactive approach to managing your blood pressure, you can significantly reduce the risk of complications and enhance your overall health and well-being.

Remember, effective blood pressure management requires a comprehensive and ongoing effort involving both self-care measures and regular communication with your healthcare provider. By prioritizing your health and implementing these preventive measures, you can take control of your blood pressure and promote a healthier future.

Now, transitioning from the discussion on the potential risks and complications associated with uncontrolled high blood pressure, let's shift our focus to a more proactive approach. One effective way to take charge of your health and reduce the risk of complications is by regularly monitoring your blood pressure.

By actively tracking your blood pressure levels, you empower yourself to make informed decisions and take necessary steps toward maintaining a healthier blood pressure range. This proactive approach enables you to stay vigilant, identify any fluctuations, and work toward achieving optimal blood pressure levels for better overall health and a reduced risk of complications. In the next chapter, we'll take a look at how you can stay in control of your health.

10

STAY ON TOP OF YOUR HEALTH

"In the long run, we shape our lives and ourselves. The process never ends until we die. And the choices we make are ultimately our own responsibility."

— ELEANOR ROOSEVELT

These profound words of Eleanor Roosevelt serve as a powerful reminder that our lives are a culmination of the choices we make. When it comes to managing high blood pressure, this truth resonates deeply. By taking an active role in our own health journey, we hold the key to influencing our well-being and paving the path toward a healthier future.

In this chapter, I will take you through the significance of self-monitoring blood pressure and its capacity to empower us in safeguarding our cardiovascular health. We will uncover the reasons why tracking our blood pressure readings goes beyond being merely beneficial—it becomes an indispensable tool in effectively managing hypertension.

Imagine the ability to monitor your blood pressure at your convenience, anytime and anywhere, liberating you from relying solely on sporadic visits to the doctor's office. By creating a personalized logbook to record your readings, you open the door to valuable insights into your blood pressure patterns, enabling you to identify triggers and make well-informed decisions regarding your lifestyle and treatment plan.

Throughout the pages ahead, I will guide you in establishing your blood pressure logbook, providing practical tips and strategies to make the process seamless and enjoyable. I will discuss various methods of measuring blood pressure, emphasizing the significance of accurate readings, and address common challenges you may encounter on this empowering journey.

Moreover, together, we will explore the numerous benefits of self-monitoring, including heightened awareness of your blood pressure fluctuations, improved communication with your healthcare provider, and the ability to detect concerning trends at their earliest stages. Armed with this knowledge, you become an active participant in your own healthcare, working hand in hand with your medical team to achieve optimal blood pressure control.

It is crucial to remember that taking charge of your blood pressure is not a fleeting commitment but a lifelong responsibility. It entails embracing your role in caring for your well-being and consciously making choices that positively impact your health. Together, let us embark on this voyage of self-monitoring and empowerment, unlocking the boundless potential to shape a future marked by improved health and unbridled happiness.

SELF-MONITORING YOUR BLOOD PRESSURE

Self-monitoring blood pressure is a critical aspect of managing hypertension and promoting overall cardiovascular health. This proactive approach empowers you to take control of your well-being, make informed decisions, and work collaboratively with healthcare professionals to achieve optimal blood pressure control.

Moreover, regularly monitoring your blood pressure at home enables you to develop a deeper comprehension of your condition and make informed choices regarding treatment and lifestyle adjustments. Some reasons why self-monitoring blood pressure is so important are:

1. Enhanced Awareness: Self-monitoring blood pressure fosters a deeper comprehension of the factors influencing blood pressure levels. Through regular tracking of readings, individuals develop a heightened awareness of how lifestyle choices, stress, and various activities impact their blood pressure. This increased awareness empowers them to make informed decisions about their daily routines and make necessary adjustments to promote better control of their blood pressure.

2. Improved Blood Pressure Management: Self-monitoring empowers individuals to actively take charge of their blood pressure on a daily basis. By consistently tracking readings, individuals can identify patterns and triggers that contribute to elevated blood pressure. Armed with this knowledge, they can make lifestyle modifications, such as adopting a healthier diet, increasing physical activity, managing stress, and adhering to prescribed medications. These proactive measures lead to better control of blood pressure and its maintenance over time.

3. Early Detection of Changes: Self-monitoring enables the timely detection of any fluctuations or sustained elevations in blood pressure. This prompt identification allows individuals to seek medical attention and necessary interventions when needed. By detecting changes early on, potential complications can be prevented or minimized, resulting in improved overall health outcomes.

4. Improved Communication with Healthcare Providers: Self-monitored blood pressure readings serve as a valuable tool for effective communication with healthcare providers. By sharing accurate and consistent data, individuals can engage in meaningful discussions about their blood pressure management.

This collaborative approach fosters a partnership between individuals and their healthcare team, ensuring treatment plans are adjusted and optimized based on real-time information. It also enables healthcare providers to make well-informed decisions regarding medication adjustments, lifestyle modifications, and other interventions for achieving optimal blood pressure control.

By incorporating self-monitoring of blood pressure into daily routines, individuals can reap numerous benefits, including heightened awareness of blood pressure triggers, improved blood pressure management, early detection of changes, and enhanced communication with healthcare providers. Actively participating in monitoring and managing blood pressure empowers individuals to take an active role in their cardiovascular health, working toward maintaining optimal well-being.

Furthermore, healthcare professionals may face challenges in determining whether your blood pressure consistently remains high or if it is only elevated during medical appointments. Several factors can contribute to fluctuations in blood pressure during a clinic visit, such as the presence of white-coat syndrome and masked hypertension.

White-coat syndrome refers to a situation where a patient experiences a temporary rise in blood pressure, specifically when it is measured in a medical setting, while their blood pressure remains normal in other environments, like their home.

Conversely, masked hypertension occurs when a patient's blood pressure appears normal during office visits, but they experience elevated blood pressure readings at other times of the day or in different settings. In both cases, the reliability of blood pressure measurements taken solely at the doctor's office becomes questionable.

The signs and symptoms of white coat syndrome include blood pressure readings that are higher than usual when measured in a medical setting, while readings outside of that environment are normal. White coat syndrome is often triggered by anxiety or stress related to medical settings or healthcare professionals. The anticipation of having blood pressure taken in a clinical setting can temporarily elevate blood pressure levels.

The signs and symptoms of masked hypertension are blood pressure readings that are normal during medical visits but elevated at other times or in different settings. Masked hypertension can be influenced by factors such as stress, physical activity, or environmental conditions that differ from the clinic setting. Monitoring blood pressure in various situations is crucial to capture the true fluctuations in blood pressure levels.

It is also important to note that higher blood pressure readings during a medical visit potentially lead to misdiagnosis or an inaccurate assessment of hypertension. This can be because engaging in physical activity shortly before a doctor's appointment can temporarily raise blood pressure due to increased heart rate and exertion. As a result, blood pressure readings taken during the visit may be elevated even if the individual's blood pressure is typically within a normal range.

There can also be an increase in blood pressure readings during a medical consultation, potentially influenced by emotional or psychological stress related to discussing health concerns. This happens when individuals are anxious or stressed about their health condition or the potential outcomes of the discussion; their blood pressure may temporarily rise. Consequently, readings during the appointment may be higher than their baseline blood pressure in a relaxed state.

These phenomena highlight the importance of self-monitoring blood pressure at home, as it provides a more comprehensive and accurate picture of your blood pressure patterns throughout the day and in various settings. By incorporating home blood pressure monitoring into your routine, you can contribute valuable data that helps healthcare professionals make well-informed decisions regarding your diagnosis, treatment, and overall management of hypertension.

MONITORING YOUR BLOOD PRESSURE AT HOME

Monitoring your blood pressure at home offers a powerful and efficient method to stay proactive about your cardiovascular well-being (American Heart Association, 2017). Regularly tracking your blood pressure readings in the comfort of your own surroundings provides invaluable insights into your blood pressure patterns, enabling you to take the necessary steps for maintaining optimal levels.

How to Utilize a Home Blood Pressure Monitor: Utilizing a home blood pressure monitor is a simple process that seamlessly fits into your routine. Begin by selecting a reliable and accurate monitor that aligns with your requirements. Adhere to the manufacturer's instructions to set up the device correctly and acquaint yourself with its features.

Properly position the cuff on your upper arm, following the provided guidelines, ensuring a snug fit without excessive tightness. Sit in a calm and relaxed environment with back support and feet flat on the floor. Rest for a few minutes prior to taking a reading, refraining from talking or moving during the measurement. Follow the device's prompts to obtain an accurate reading, and record the results in your blood pressure logbook or smartphone app.

Understanding Your Numbers: Understanding the meaning behind your blood pressure numbers is crucial for effective monitoring. Blood pressure is represented by two values:

systolic pressure (the top number) and diastolic pressure (the bottom number).

The American Heart Association defines normal blood pressure as below 120/80 mmHg. Readings between 120–129 (systolic) and below 80 (diastolic) indicate elevated blood pressure. Hypertension is categorized into two stages: stage 1 (130–139/80–89) and stage 2 (140 or higher/90 or higher). Familiarize yourself with these numbers and consult your healthcare provider for personalized guidance and target ranges based on your medical history and risk factors.

Responding to High Blood Pressure Readings: Obtaining a high blood pressure reading at home should not cause panic. Take a deep breath and remain composed, remembering that individual readings can fluctuate throughout the day due to various factors.

If consistently recording high readings, it is crucial to reach out to your healthcare provider to discuss the results and seek further evaluation. They can determine if lifestyle adjustments, medication modifications, or additional tests are necessary.

Selecting a Home Blood Pressure Monitor: Choosing the right home blood pressure monitor is essential for accurate and dependable readings. Consider factors such as cuff size, ease of use, display readability, and validated accuracy.

Seek monitors validated by reputable organizations like the Association for the Advancement of Medical Instrumentation (AAMI) or the British Hypertension Society (BHS). Consult with your healthcare provider for recommendations regarding specific models or brands that suit your needs.

Left-Arm vs. Right-Arm Blood Pressure: When monitoring your blood pressure at home, establish consistency in arm selection. Both the left and right arms can provide accurate readings, but it is recommended to consistently use either arm for monitoring. This ensures measurement consistency and facilitates easier comparison of readings over time.

Monitoring your blood pressure at home places you in control of your health. By following proper techniques, comprehending your numbers, seeking professional guidance when required, and selecting a reliable monitor, you can effectively track your blood pressure and work toward maintaining optimal cardiovascular health.

KEEPING A BLOOD PRESSURE LOGBOOK

Keeping a blood pressure logbook is an invaluable tool for effectively managing your blood pressure and gaining deeper insights into your cardiovascular well-being. This logbook acts as a complete record of your blood pressure readings, enabling you to monitor trends, identify patterns, and make informed decisions concerning your lifestyle and treatment regimen. Here are the essential components of a blood pressure logbook:

1. Date and Time of Readings: Recording the date and time of each blood pressure reading is crucial for tracking your progress over time. This information allows you to observe any changes or trends that may occur throughout the day or over extended periods.

2. Systolic and Diastolic Blood Pressure Numbers: The logbook should include sections to record the systolic and diastolic blood pressure numbers for each reading. The systolic pressure represents the force exerted on artery walls when the heart contracts, while the diastolic pressure reflects the pressure when the heart is at rest between beats. Monitoring both values provides a comprehensive understanding of your blood pressure levels.

3. Heart Rate: In addition to blood pressure readings, monitoring your heart rate is valuable for assessing your cardiovascular health. Note your heart rate alongside each blood pressure reading to monitor any changes or irregularities.

4. Medications Taken: Allocate a section in the logbook to document the medications you have taken before each blood pressure reading. This information helps you evaluate the effectiveness of your medications and their impact on your blood pressure levels.

5. Notes on Symptoms or Lifestyle Changes: Develop a habit of jotting down any symptoms or lifestyle changes that may influence your blood pressure. For example, if you experience stress, engage in physical activity, consume caffeine, or make significant dietary changes, record these factors. These notes assist in identifying potential triggers or patterns that affect your blood pressure readings.

By consistently maintaining a blood pressure logbook, you possess a comprehensive record that enables you and your healthcare provider to review your progress, make informed adjustments to your treatment plan, and develop personalized strategies for effectively managing your blood pressure.

Tips for accuracy and consistency

1. Choose a Reliable Blood Pressure Monitor: Invest in a high-quality blood pressure monitor that has been validated and approved by reputable organizations like the Association for the Advancement of Medical Instrumentation (AAMI) or the British Hypertension Society (BHS). Regularly calibrate and maintain the monitor to ensure accurate readings.

2. Maintain a Consistent Measurement Schedule: Establish a fixed routine for measuring your blood pressure. Aim to take readings at the same time each day to minimize variations caused by daily fluctuations. Recommended times include mornings before taking medications and evenings before bedtime.

3. Use a Standardized Recording System: Keep a standardized record sheet or utilize a digital blood pressure tracking app. This promotes consistency in documenting your blood pressure readings, making it easier to identify trends and share the information with your healthcare provider. Include essential details such as date, time, blood pressure readings, heart rate, and any relevant notes.

4. Select a Quiet Environment for Measurements: Choose a calm and quiet location for taking blood pressure readings. Minimize distractions and external influences that could impact your blood pressure, such as noise or interruptions. Sit in a comfortable chair with proper back support and ensure your feet are flat on the floor, as this helps obtain accurate readings.

5. Record Each Reading Promptly: After measuring your blood pressure, immediately record the results in your log sheet or digital tracking app. This ensures precise and timely documentation, reducing the risk of errors or misinterpretation. Avoid delays in recording to maintain the accuracy of your log.

6. Share Your Log with Your Healthcare Provider: During check-ups or appointments, share your blood pressure log sheet or digital records with your healthcare provider. This enables them to review your progress, identify any concerning patterns, and make informed decisions about your treatment plan. Take the opportunity to discuss any questions or concerns you have regarding your readings to receive guidance and clarification.

By adhering to these guidelines for accuracy and consistency in blood pressure monitoring, you can rely on reliable and comparable readings. This empowers you to track your blood pressure effectively and facilitates productive discussions with your healthcare provider for optimal management of your cardiovascular health.

BLOOD PRESSURE LOGBOOK

Here is a sample logbook page designed for tracking your blood pressure measurements at home. This page offers designated spaces to record essential information, including the date, time, systolic and diastolic blood pressure readings, as well as heart rate.

By diligently completing this logbook page, you can effectively monitor your cardiovascular well-being, detect trends, and identify any recurring patterns. Remember to employ a trustworthy blood pressure monitor and adhere to correct measurement techniques.

Regularly sharing this logbook with your healthcare provider encourages fruitful discussions and enables informed decisions regarding your treatment plan. Embrace control over your health by utilizing this logbook to maintain a comprehensive overview of your blood pressure measurements.

Remember, by assuming command over your blood pressure through self-monitoring and making adjustments to your lifestyle, you have the power to substantially diminish the likelihood of complications and enhance your overall well-being. Through a suitable blend of medications, self-care practices, and consistent monitoring, you can effectively manage your blood pressure and enjoy an improved quality of life.

Time	Blood Pressure (mm Hg)		Heart Rate	Comments (e.g., activity change, diet change, medication change)
	Systolic (upper #)	Diastolic (lower #)		

CONCLUSION

Managing high blood pressure effectively can result in notable enhancements in health results. According to research by Yang et al. (2017), it was revealed that the utilization of medication and modifications in one's lifestyle, like shedding excess weight, engaging in physical activity, and employing stress management techniques, can lower the chances of developing heart disease, stroke, and other complications linked to elevated blood pressure The study also revealed that insufficient control of blood pressure was linked to weight gain, lack of physical activity, and excessive salt consumption.

This information emphasizes the significance of assuming responsibility for managing your blood pressure and collaborating closely with healthcare professionals to create a successful treatment strategy. By implementing a suitable combination of medications, lifestyle adjustments, and regular monitoring, individuals can substantially diminish their chances of experiencing complications and enjoy a healthier and more energetic life.

Don't wait for a health scare to take charge of your blood pressure. Start making small adjustments to your lifestyle today, such as incorporating exercise and adopting a heart-healthy diet. Work collaboratively with your healthcare providers to develop an effective treatment plan that suits your needs.

By doing so, you can significantly decrease the likelihood of heart disease, stroke, and other complications. Remember, taking control of your health is an ongoing journey. Stay proactive by monitoring your blood pressure regularly, staying updated on the latest research and treatment options, and seeking support from healthcare professionals and loved ones. Maintain your progress and embrace a healthy, happy life.

PAY IT FORWARD

WANT TO HELP OTHERS?

As we've said, knowledge is power… and this is your chance to spread it to help others.

Simply by sharing your honest opinion of this book and a little about your own experience, you'll show new readers that they're not alone and there's guidance out there to help them take control.

If you found this book valuable and insightful, I would greatly appreciate it if you could take a moment to leave a review. Thank you for your support and sharing your thoughts!

Follow Dr. Ashley Sullivan, PharmD on Facebook

And on her website **ashleysullivanonline.com**

Scan the QR code below

REFERENCES

5 Steps to Quit Smoking. (2018). Www.heart.org. https://www.heart.org/en/healthy-living/healthy-lifestyle/quit-smoking-tobacco/5-steps-to-quit-smoking.

Alcohol and Heart Health: Separating Fact from Fiction. (n.d.). Www.hopkinsmedicine.org. https://www.hopkinsmedicine.org/health/wellness-and-prevention/alcohol-and-heart-health-separating-fact-from-fiction.

American Heart Association. (2017). Monitoring Your Blood Pressure at Home. Www.heart.org. https://www.heart.org/en/health-topics/high-blood-pressure/understanding-blood-pressure-readings/monitoring-your-blood-pressure-at-home.

Amin, M. (2020, January 9). Supplements vs Food: The Truth Behind Multi-Vitamins and Eating Right. Regenerate Medical Concierge. https://regeneratemedicalconcierge.com/supplements-vs-food-the-truth-behind-multi-vitamins-and-eating-right/.

Anderson, J. W., Liu, C., & Kryscio, R. J. (2008). Blood Pressure Response to Transcendental Meditation: A Meta-analysis. American Journal of Hypertension, 21(3), 310–316. https://doi.org/10.1038/ajh.2007.65.

Beckerman, J. (2021, September). The Link Between Drinking Alcohol and Heart Disease? WebMD. https://www.webmd.com/heart-disease/heart-disease-alcohol-your-heart

CDC. (2017, June 30). Benefits of Quitting. Centers for Disease Control and Prevention. https://www.cdc.gov/tobacco/quit_smoking/how_to_quit/benefits/index.htm.

BSc, K. G. (2023, May 17). Mediterranean Diet 101: A Meal Plan and Beginner's Guide. Healthline. https://www.healthline.com/nutrition/mediterranean-diet-meal-plan#menu-and-recipes.

Carol Dersarkissian. (2021). Slideshow: What Happens to Your Body When You Quit Smoking.WebMD.https://www.webmd.com/smoking-cessation/ss/slideshow-effects-of-quitting-smoking.

CDC. (2020, November 9). 5 Surprising Facts About High Blood Pressure |

cdc.gov. Centers for Disease Control and Prevention. https://www.cdc.gov/bloodpressure/5_surprising_facts.htm.

Cleveland Clinic. (2022, January 7). Blood Pressure: Treatments. Cleveland Clinic. https://my.clevelandclinic.org/health/diseases/17649-blood-pressure.

Contributors, W. E. (2023, April 29). Complementary vs. Alternative Medicine: What's the Difference? WebMD. https://www.webmd.com/balance/complementary-vs-alternative-medicine

Crouch, M. (2020, July 28). 7 Ways to Overcome Your Fitness Fears. AARP. https://www.aarp.org/health/healthy-living/info-2020/overcoming-fitness-fears.html.

D. Fryar, C., Ostchega, Y., M. Hales, C., Zhang, G., & Kruszon-Moran, D. (2019). Products - Data Briefs - Number 289 - October 2017. https://www.cdc.gov/nchs/products/databriefs/db289.htm.

DASH diet: Sample menus. (2023, May 31). Mayo Clinic. https://www.mayoclinic.org/healthy-lifestyle/nutrition-and-healthy-eating/in-depth/dash-diet/art-20047110.

Dekker, A. (2021, July 26). What are the effects of alcohol on the brain? Scientific American. https://www.scientificamerican.com/article/what-are-the-effects-of-a/

Eskarda. (2022, February 22). 6 Yoga Poses for High Blood Pressure. Yoga Journal. https://www.yogajournal.com/poses/yoga-by-benefit/high-blood-pressure/yoga-for-high-blood-pressure/.

Exercise: A drug-free approach to lowering high blood pressure. (2022, November 10). Mayo Clinic. https://www.mayoclinic.org/diseases-conditions/high-blood-pressure/in-depth/high-blood-pressure/art-20045206.

Francis, M. (2021, April 29). If slightly high blood pressure doesn't respond to lifestyle change, medication can help. American Heart Association. https://newsroom.heart.org/news/if-slightly-high-blood-pressure-doesnt-respond-to-lifestyle-change-medication-can-help.

Harvard Health. (2020, July 4). 11 ways to curb your drinking. Harvard Health. https://www.health.harvard.edu/staying-healthy/11-ways-to-curb-your-drinking.

Harvard Health Publishing. (2021). The benefits of do-it-yourself blood pressure monitoring. Harvard Health. https://www.health.harvard.edu/heart-health/the-benefits-of-do-it-yourself-blood-pressure-monitoring.

Harvard School of Public Health. (2016, April 12). Healthy Weight. The Nutrition Source. https://www.hsph.harvard.edu/nutritionsource/healthy-weight/.

Hitti, M. (2013, August 22). 10 Relaxation Techniques That Zap Stress Fast. WebMD; WebMD. https://www.webmd.com/balance/guide/blissing-out-10-relaxation-techniques-reduce-stress-spot.

Houston, M. C., & Harper, K. J. (2008). Potassium, Magnesium, and Calcium: Their Role in Both the Cause and Treatment of Hypertension. The Journal of Clinical Hypertension, 10(7), 3–11. https://doi.org/10.1111/j.1751-7176.2008.08575.x.

Hypertension Prevalence in the U.S. | Million Hearts®. (2023, May 12). Centers for Disease Control and Prevention. https://millionhearts.hhs.gov/data-reports/hypertension-prevalence.html.

L. Bhatt, D. (2022, May 1). Yoga and high blood pressure. Harvard Health. https://www.health.harvard.edu/heart-health/yoga-and-high-blood-pressure.

Landry, J. (2023, January 31). *72+ best hypertension quotes and sayings for inspiration (2023)*. Respiratory Therapy Zone. https//www.respiratorytherapyzone.com/hypertension-quotes/

Landsbergis, P., Diez-Roux, A. V., Fujishiro, K., Baron, S., Kaufman, J. D., Meyer, J. S., Koutsouras, G. W., Shimbo, D., Shrager, S., Stukovsky, K. H., & Szklo, M. (2015). Job Strain, Occupational Category, Systolic Blood Pressure, and Hypertension Prevalence. Journal of Occupational and Environmental Medicine, 57(11), 1178–1184. https://doi.org/10.1097/jom.0000000000000533.

Mawer, R. (2020, February 28). 17 Proven Tips to Sleep Better at Night. Healthline. https://www.healthline.com/nutrition/17-tips-to-sleep-better.

Mayo Clinic. (2015). Exercise: A drug-free approach to lowering high blood pressure. Mayo Clinic. https://www.mayoclinic.org/diseases-conditions/high-blood-pressure/in-depth/high-blood-pressure/art-20045206.

Mayo Clinic. (2021). How high blood pressure can affect your body. Mayo Clinic. https://www.mayoclinic.org/diseases-conditions/high-blood-pressure/in-depth/high-blood-pressure/art-20045868#

Miller, D. (2021). Complementary and Alternative Treatments for Hypertension. https://ruralhealth.und.edu/assets/4283-18665/treatments-for-hypertension.pdf

National Institute on Aging. (2021). Vascular Dementia: Causes, Symptoms, and Treatments. National Institute on Aging. https://www.nia.nih.gov/health/vascular-dementia.

NHS. (2019, February 11). Intensive blood pressure control may lessen cognitive loss. National Institutes of Health (NIH). https://www.nih.gov/news-events/nih-research-matters/intensive-blood-pressure-control-may-lessen-cognitive-loss#

Porter, E. (2017, November 14). Famous Faces of Heart Disease. Healthline. https://www.healthline.com/health/celebrities-with-heart-disease#david-letterman

Publishing, H. H. (2020, June 14). Meditation and a relaxation technique to lower blood pressure. Harvard Health. https://www.health.harvard.edu/heart-health/meditation-and-a-relaxation-technique-to-lower-blood-pressure.

Richter, A. (2020, December 23). 14 Supplements That May Help Lower Blood Pressure. Healthline. https://www.healthline.com/nutrition/supplements-lower-blood-pressure,

Salvetti, A., Brogi, G., Di Legge, V., & Bernini, G. P. (1993). The inter-relationship between insulin resistance and hypertension. Drugs, 46 Suppl 2, 149–159. https://doi.org/10.2165/00003495-199300462-00024.

Schneider, J. K., Reangsing, C., & Willis, D. G. (2022). Effects of Transcendental Meditation on Blood Pressure. Journal of Cardiovascular Nursing, 37(3), E11–E21. https://doi.org/10.1097/jcn.0000000000000849.

Suni, E. (2021, March 10). How Much Sleep Do We Really Need? | National Sleep Foundation (A. Singh, Ed.). Sleep Foundation. https://www.sleepfoundation.org/how-sleep-works/how-much-sleep-do-we-really-need.

Tackling, G., & Borhade, M. B. (2022). Hypertensive Heart Disease. PubMed; StatPearls Publishing. https://www.ncbi.nlm.nih.gov/books/NBK539800/#:~:text=Hypertension%20disrupts%20the%20endothelial%20system.

U.S. Food and Drug Administration. (2022, June 2). FDA 101: Dietary Supplements. U.S. Food and Drug Administration. https://www.fda.gov/consumers/consumer-updates/fda-101-dietary-supplements.

W. Smith, M. (2021, September 20). Slideshow: 20 Foods That Can Save Your Heart. WebMD. https://www.webmd.com/heart-disease/ss/slideshow-foods-to-save-your-heart.

Wein, H. (2017, September 8). Understanding Health Risks. NIH News in Health. https://newsinhealth.nih.gov/2016/10/understanding-health-risks.

Why High Blood Pressure is a "Silent Killer." (2023, May 31). www.heart.org. https://www.heart.org/en/health-topics/high-blood-pressure/why-high-blood-pressure-is-a-silent-killer.

World Health Organization: WHO & World Health Organization: WHO. (2023). Hypertension. www.who.int. https://www.who.int/news-room/fact-sheets/detail/hypertension#

Yang, M. H., Kang, S. Y., Lee, J. A., Kim, Y. S., Sung, E. J., Lee, K.-Y., Kim, J.-S., Oh, H. J., Kang, H. C., & Lee, S. Y. (2017). The Effect of Lifestyle Changes on Blood Pressure Control among Hypertensive Patients. Korean Journal of Family Medicine, 38(4), 173. https://doi.org/10.4082/kjfm.2017.38.4.173.

www.ingramcontent.com/pod-product-compliance
Lightning Source LLC
Chambersburg PA
CBHW070607030426
42337CB00020B/3704